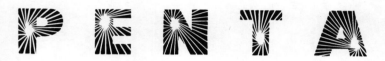

MANUAL

WALDO VIEIRA, M.D.

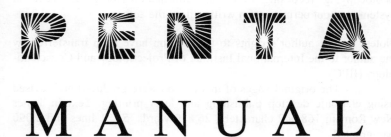

PENTA MANUAL

PERSONAL ENERGETIC TASK

Translators:
Kevin de La Tour
Simone de La Tour

Proofreaders:
Cecilia Finkelstein
Pamela Hughes

First Edition in English

Rio de Janeiro, RJ – Brazil
International Institute of Projectiology and Conscientiology
1996

Notes: - The author's rights to this edition have been transferred by the author to the International Institute of Projectiology and Conscientiology (IIPC).
    - The original pages of this edition were produced and revised using eletronic desktop publishing and laser printing. Text in Times New Roman; 168,642 characters; 26,880 words; 5,221 lines and 2,090 paragraphs).

Cover: Fernando Alberto Santos & Günther Kismann
Photo: Geysa Adnet
Printing and biding: OESP Gráfica

Card Catalog Information prepared by
International Institute of Projectiology and Conscientiology (IIPC)
Center of Information and Documentation

Vieira, Waldo, 1932 –

V658p   Penta manual: personal energetic task / Waldo Vieira. –
         1ª Edition in English – Rio de Janeiro: International Institute of Projectiology and Conscientiology, 1996.
         148 p.

         1. Conscientiology. 2. Projectiology. I. Title

ISBN 85.86019.16.X   CDD 133

IIPC - International Institute of Projectiology and Conscientiology
R. Visconde de Pirajá, 572 / 6° andar – Ipanema – Rio de Janeiro – RJ – Brasil – CEP 22410-002
Fone (5521) 512.9229 – Fax (5521) 512.4735
Caixa Postal 70.000 – CEP 22422-970
Internet: E-mail: iip@ax.ibase.org.br
         Home Page: http://www.ibase.org.br/~iip

TABLE OF CONTENTS

INTRODUCTION

Manual. This volume is the *"book about penta"* that many colleagues, collaborators, energizers, *projectiologists* and *conscientiologists* (students of *Projectiology* and *Conscientiology*) have been requesting from this author over the last 2 decades.

Research. The *Manual* was reorganized from: personal notes dating back to 1950; research with men and women practitioners of the *personal energetic task*; and through questions and answers gathered in the *"Courses on Penta"*, given recently through the educational programs of the International Institute of Projectiology, in various locations.

Para-technology. This book, dedicated to the execution of projective, psychic, transcendent experiments, fits in an area of leading-edge highly *para-technological consciousness* research.

Variables. You who are being exposed to this subject for the first time, *should not waste time* with this practical manual *if you do not accept*, with lethal surety, the following 5 variables:

1. *Consciential energy.* The existence – well established by yourself – of *consciential (personal) energy*, beyond the nerve impulses of the human body.
2. Animism. Benign, evolutionary animic (self-produced) manifestations, beyond belief systems, delirium and folkloric traditions.
3. Psychic capacity. Healthy *psychic manifestations* (mediumistic, interdimensional or *paranormal*).
4. *Interassistentiality.* The evolutionary necessity for *human consciousnesses* to assist each other through logical, just and mature *interassistential works*.
5. *Interdimensionality. Interconsciential* communication between the many *intraphysical* (physical) and *extraphysical* (non-physical) dimensions.

Resources. Logically, it would be better, in the case of not agreeing with all the above items, to leave this subject aside until you have already experienced, for yourself, the above issues calmly and without the disturbance of controversy, as a part of an inevitably discerning, cultural, social, *intraphysical* microminority.

Predisposition. This volume of experiments does not evidence any pretense by the author-informer to persuade anyone. It is only a practical codification for *those who are predisposed to the theme.* That is why , if you do not fit within these conditions, the most intelligent thing to do is to postpone your assistential, energetic and *consciential* development for a later date or even for the *intraphysical* directives of another *existential program*, a better *intermissive course* and *another soma* down the line, at a new stage in the procession of successive human lives.

Truth. *Consciential maturity* shows logically that every leading-edge relative truth, when of a greater nature, is preceded by 3 occurrences of discernment, far surpassing good will and good intention:

1. Entropy. *First* provokes an expansion of your localized entropy (self-disorganization, personal indiscipline), in order to *later* diminish entropy in general.
2. Stress. *First* generates the uncomfortable, pathological stress of a growing crisis in the *multi-dimensional here-and-now*, in order to *later* generate healthy, liberating, personal stress.
3. Neophobia. *First* irritates, in the condition of instinctive neophobia (fear of the new and vanguard), to *later* increase one's evolved neophilia or the desire for and gratification from evolutionary discoveries, the animus and motivation towards disciplined self-awareness.

Precedence. Penta is the most effective and only technique known and used by this author – in his approximately halfcentury of psychic experiences – and now technically codified, to maintain the human being (*intraphysical consciousness*) connected to his or her *extraphysical, evolutionary precedence* (the extraphysical community you resided in before intraphysical rebirth) beyond the terrestrial troposphere, without being subjected to spurious effects from any temporal or *intraphysical* causes.

WE LIVE AS ANTS ON THE SKIN OF AN ORANGE THAT IS PLANET EARTH.

Soma. In our everyday life, we generally do not think about our real precedence, where we are from, what we are doing or should be doing here, and where we are going with our efforts, lives or destinies, after the inevitable deactivation of the human body.

Exit. We have to *intraphysically* and *extraphysically* leave the surface of this planet in order to sustain the evolution of each and all of us, at our current evolutionary level.

Pre-kundalini. When man arrived on the Moon, the first thing he did was to place his *pre-kundalini* (sole-chakra) on the surface or *skin* of the satellite, allowing the celebrated photo of the astronaut's footstep on this terrestrial satellite.

Ants. The astronaut's footprint is a perfect example that we have the tendency to live in a condition of *tropospheric consciousness, as ants on an orange.*

Cosmos. That this volume helps you to leave this *orange* and travel into the immense *orange grove* of the Cosmos, through *maxi-fraternity (mega-brotherhood),* is the hope of .

the Author

1. DEFINITIONS

Definition. *Penta* (*personal energetic task*) is an individual, assistential transmission of *consciential* (personal) *energy*, programmed for a certain hour in the day of a *human consciousness*, assisted by one or more *Helpers*, in waking state; directly to ill or deficient that are intangible and invisible to typical human vision; or to ill or deficient projected *intraphysical consciousnesses*, whether close-by or at a distance.

Synonymy. The following 9 expressions characterize the practice of *penta:*

1. *Mega-challenge* for the human being.

2. *Energetic pass* (transmission) given to an *unknown patient.*

3. *Passes-to-the-dark.*

4. Solitary *psychic passivity.*

5. *Unitary psychological group therapy.*

6. *Assistential benign semi-possession.*

7. Service of *energetic compensation.*

8. Individual *energetic-animic-psychic session.*

9. *Psychic* or mediumistic *session* of me alone.

THE PRACTICE OF PENTA IS A NON-REMUNERATED ENERGETIC--ASSISTENTIAL SERVICE.

Link. The *personal energetic task* is based on a *consciential link* between the *human mini-piece* (man or woman) and the multi-dimensional, *assistential maxi-mechanism* (team having its origin in the greater *extraphysical* dimension).

THE PENTA PRACTITIONER IS AN INTERDIMENSIONAL AXLE.

Denominations. S/he who develops the *daily personal energetic task*, in the manner analyzed in this volume, generally receives 6 diverse denominations:

1. Daily *interconsciential assistant.*

2. *Consciential energizer.*

3. Self-aware *consciential epicenter.*

4. *Passes-to-the-dark practitioner.*

5. *Interdimensional axle.*

6. *Penta practitioner.*

Millstone. We must try to logically understand that the *penta practitioner*, in the position of *interconsciential epicenter*, is the *millstone of the mill* used in the work of the assistential, multi-dimensional, energetic maxi-mechanism.

2. HISTORY OF PENTA

History. *Penta*, in its empirical, fetal, instinctive form, devoid of technique, has existed since time immemorial in a sketchy form among those *human consciousnesses* aware of multidimensionality. These practices have existed in a form both aggravated and *polluted* by the intrusion of mysticism, archetypes, *brain washings, intraphysical* conditionings, sacralizations, human insufficiencies, and all manner of cultural and social repressions.

Launching. Penta was actually launched to the greater public in 1966, according to the registry made on page 958 of the book *"700 Conscientiology Experiments".*

Epistemology. Only *Projectiology* and *Conscientiology*, from a technical and practical point of view, and an epistemological point of view, respectively, have codified penta's practices in a productive, dynamic and rational manner.

Religion. *Penta* exists in order to substitute and, with time, definitively eliminate the need for unconscious or instinctive adoration of faith, belief or any type of *religion* and its essential practices (religious vows, religious professionalisms, and others) on the part of the *intraphysical consciousness.*

The "reconnection" of a *consciousness* is made with its precedence and not with a supposed "God" or primary cause. The creation and the Creator become secondary. This is unimportant for the evolutionary immediatist of the *multi-dimensional here-and-now.* The *penta* practitioner does not have a lucid, evolutionary, utilitarian, pragmatic need for concepts about God, creation or Creator, in our current level of *consciential* progress.

Confidence. Penta dispenses with prayers, orations, mysticism, promises and abstruse rituals of all types. All penta practitioners depend on personal organization, self-sufficiency, perseverance and confidence in the *Helpers* responsible for the mechanism of installed *interconsciential* and multi-dimensional assistance.

PENTA IS AN IDEAL SUBSTITUTION FOR SOCIAL ASSISTANCE.

Assistentiality. The fundamental assistance of *penta* includes 2 categories of Helpers: the *Helper* of the penta *practitioner* and the *Helper* of *those being assisted* through *penta*.

Objectives. The penta practitioner has more far reaching objectives than his or her personal interests. S/he seeks to master his or her *consciential energies*, not in order to be a "great evolved *consciousness*", but to perform efficient assistentiality between *consciousnesses*.

Inevitability. Given everything that we will be analyzing, any *consciousness* can easily reach the conclusion that *penta* is an irreplaceable and inevitable process, on the part of the *human consciousness*, after reaching a certain level of evolution.

Superintendence. There are no codes, statutes, laws, commercial firms, industries, public ministries, or human institutions that superintend or fiscally regulate the practice of penta. Its roots are *extraphysical* or multi-dimensional.

PENTA IS AN EXTRA-HUMAN PRACTICE OF INTRAPHYSICAL CONSCIOUSNESS.

Extra-human. There are other *extra-human practices* that no human organ or institution, ministry or autocracy, charges taxes on or fiscally regulates. Following are 5 examples:

1. Execution of one's *existential program*.

2. *Extraphysical clinic*.

3. Energetic-animic-psychic *signals*.

4. *Vibrational state*

5. Greater *conscious projection*.

Cosmoethic. One's experience of the cosmoethic – innate in the individual, through their relationship with the Helpers – is the supervisory agent of the practices and natural development of *penta*.

3. INTRAPHYSICAL CONSCIOUSNESSES

Facets. The various facets, strong traits and weak traits of *intraphysical consciousnesses* can be classified into 2 basic groups, each having 23 types, relative to *penta:*

PRO-PENTA INTRAPHYSICAL CONSCIOUSNESSES	ANTI-PENTA INTRAPHYSICAL CONSCIOUSNESSES
Homo amicus	Homo animalis
Homo arbiter	Homo artifex
Homo divinans	Homo bellicosus
Homo duplex	Homo civicus
Homo fraternus	Homo competitor
Homo universalis	Homo submissus
Homo habilis	Homo erectus
Homo socialis	Homo supersticiosus
Homo humanus	Homo eroticus
Homo idealis	Homo theatrallis
Homo informaticus	Homo faber
Homo intellegens	Homo genuflexus
Homo invulgaris	Homo loquax
Homo laboriosus	Homo hostilis
Homo logicus	Homo ludens
Homo pacificus	Homo maniacus
Homo sapiens	Homo mythicus
Homo projectius	Homo mercuralis
Homo technicus	Homo viator
Homo psychicus	Homo politicus
Homo sanus	Homo signifex
Homo sapientor	Homo stultus
Homo spiritualis	Homo sportivus

ARE YOU A PRO-PENTA OR ANTI-
-PENTA HUMAN CONSCIOUSNESS?

4. PARADOXES

Paradoxes. Among the greatest demonstrations of the *intra-physical consciousness* self-sufficiency, we can point out the following 4 *paradoxical consciential techniques,* as they are based on an inevitable interdependence with other *consciousnesses:*

1. *Penta,* or *personal energetic task,* a daily practice that depends on the *Helpers.*

2. *Extraphysical clinic* of *interconsciential* and interdimensional assistance, the advanced functioning of which also depends on the *Helpers.*

3. *Existential completism* (the condition of having completed one's *existential program* – personal task or mission) regarding our *existential program,* the achievement of which depends on our general relationship with our *evolutionary group* or karmic group.

4. *Existential moratorium* (an extension of intraphysical life), a condition which depends on the *Evolutionary Orientor* (Helper who oversees the existential tasks of a number of individuals), to a certain degree.

5. COMPARISONS

Fundamentals. In this chapter we will seek to establish some associations between ideas and make didactic comparisons in order to clarify and better define the fundamentals of the practice of *penta.*

Cosmo-consciousness. The physical and psychic state of the *penta* practitioner, during the assistential energetic transmissions, can be compared to a condition of *cosmo-consciousness* (state of total expansion of *consciousness*) while *in* the waking state.

Assistentiality. The percentage of possible *interconsciential* energetic assistance – through the use of *consciential energy* – that certain conditions of affinity permit is clearly quite diverse. Following is an example in order of increasing assistentiality:

1. *Incomplete couple*   =   X %
2. *Intimate couple*   =   2X %
3. Practitioner-Helper connection   =   3X %

Duo. The above illustration of *interconsciential* connections emphatically shows the critical superiority of commitment between the *penta practitioner* and the assistential *Helper* (2 *professionals*) over the evolved condition of the *evolutionary duo* (*literally*, always 2 lovers).

Multi-dimensionality. Following are 9 points of evidence regarding multi-dimensionality or interdimensionality *among consciential dimensions*:

1. Maturity. The greatest *consciential maturity* is interdimensional.

2. *Cosmoethic.* The *cosmoethic* is interdimensional.

3. Charisma. The maximal, transcendent charisma (*consciential energy*) is interdimensional.

4. *Projectability.* All *projectability* of *consciousness* is interdimensional.

5. Universalism. All pure universalism having a greater vision of *consciousness* is interdimensional.

6. *Clarification task*. The *assistential task of clarification* opens the doors of interdimensional life to the aware *intraphysical consciousness*.

7. *Poly-karmality*. Evolved *poly-karmality*, being more advanced than *ego-karma* and *group-karma*, is *interdimensional (Ego-karma* relates to individual karma; *group-karma* relates to the karma of one's *evolutionary groups*; poly-karma is centered in an experience of cosmic *maxi-fraternity)*.

8. *Serenism*. *Serenism* that is incorporated into one's daily life is interdimensional.

9. *Penta*. The daily *personal energetic task* is interdimensional.

Availability. *Penta* represents maximum *personal* availability for *whatever may happen* in terms of *offering yourself* completely in regards to *interconsciential* and multi-dimensional assistance. *Penta* is a definitive, standardized, regular obligation that continues for the rest of one's human life.

Course. The *course Extension in Conscientiology and Projectiology 2* (ECP2), given by the International Institute of Projectiology, is a preparation for the exercise of *penta* for the rest of one's human existence.

THERE IS NO LOGICAL PLACE FOR SELF-CORRUPTION – ESPECIALLY IN PENTA.

Self-corruption. *Self-corruption* can have no place in the healthy, *cosmoethical* practice of *penta*. When this occurs, the practitioner is subject to conscious victimization by his or her personal, group or task-related *intruders* (imbalanced nonphysical *consciousnesses*).

Will. In theory, and with the natural realism with which the subjects in this *manual* are exposed, all persons, men and women, have some type of *intruder(s)*. Unfortunately, no one living on the face of this planet, up until now, is exempt from this uncomfortable condition. Given this fact, the choice to operate in a *positive* or *negative* manner is always a function of the will of the *penta practitioner.*

Helper. Unfortunately, at certain levels of self-corruption, a *Helper* can do nothing to assistentially and *cosmoethically* intercede between the practitioner and his or her *intruders.* At times they can only *strategically remove themselves,* waiting for a *better time to assist,* and leave the scenario because *they do not find it agreeable.* Unfortunately.

Phase. The pathological condition of conscious self-corruption becomes more *acute and dramatic* during the first 6-month phase of the beginning *penta* practitioner.

Existence. Each penta session is like one lucid, temporary, *multi-dimensional, assistential existence* of 50 minutes, that is experienced every day, for the rest of the course of one's *intraphysical life.*

PENTA DEMANDS THAT THE PRACTITIONER NOT THINK BADLY OF ANYONE.

Hygiene. Without discarding one's scientific and *cosmoethical* self-, hetero- and omni-questioning nature, the practitioner must choose to see, with all sincerity, the *better side* of persons, *extraphysical consciousnesses,* ambiances, objects, ideas and institutions, in order to *help* all involved. This must be done *neither by sugar-coating things,* nor in a manner of demagogic consolation. This is the *cosmoethic hygiene* of the *penta practitioner.*

Affection. The *penta practitioner* will, with time, inevitably come to like or have a much greater spontaneous, real affection and fraternal love for his or her fellow beings, or rather, *intraphysical* and *extraphysical humanity.*

Transcendence. The assistential occurrences during the practice of *penta* are too didactic, evolved and transcendent to allow the *intraphysical consciousness* to become complacent in a mediocrity that is still subhuman or submissive to the *belly-brain* (*abdominal sub-brain*: a parody of the natural, encephalic brain). *Consciential epicenter.* With the development of his or her exercises over time, the *penta practitioner* becomes a veteran – or a *consciential epicenter* – of *interconsciential* assistance through the establishment of the following 6 conditions:

1. Security. Point of self-assured security.
2. Support. Point of interconsciential support.
3. Assistance. Multi-faceted energetic assistance.
4. Pole. Pole of conscious *de-intrusion* (extraphysical cleansing of unbalanced non-physical consciousnesses).
5. Mini-piece. Conscious *mini-*piece of an assistential multi-dimensional *maxi-*mechanism.
6. Ambassador. *Intra*physical ambassador of the *extra*physical *Evolutionary Orientor.*

THE EVOLUTIONARY ORIENTOR IS THE EXTRAPHYSICAL SUPER-HELPER OF THE KARMIC GROUP.

6. PENTA TECHNIQUE

Preparation. In preparation for penta you, as a psychic *intraphysical consciousness*, intraphysically alone, make yourself comfortable on your bed, preferably in the dark. Relax, calm your mind, and become psychically and physically passive to the extraphysical Helper, who is a specialist in *interconsciential* assistance.

Semi-possession. You will then be overcome by the phenomenon of *benign or healthy, interconsciential possession or semi-possession* for the transmission of *consciential energies.* This will occur with you, the practitioner, seated in bed, reclining in a chair, or standing up.

Monitoring. This *benign semi-possession* allows the maintenance of constant *extraphysical monitoring* of the *penta practitioner* on the part of the *Helper(s).*

Place. *Penta* should be practiced in a *dark room* with the doors and windows closed, with no noisy instruments around. Penta should always be performed in the same place.

Bedroom. The *bedroom*, in many cases, is the best place to practice *penta.*

Living room. The *living room* should be avoided for the execution of penta, given its *public atmosphere* and lack of privacy.

Bathroom. The *bathroom* is obviously not an appropriate place to perform penta. It would not be polite to receive a *Helper* – *one of the most illustrious visitors* that you receive in your home – in the bathroom, even if it is spotlessly clean.

Exclusivity. If you can, reserve a portion of or space in your house or apartment exclusively for the practice of *penta.* This is ideal, but impractical for most.

Precognitarium. Penta that is developed in a *precognitarium* (space that is designed to engender *precognitive projections*) obviously dynamizes the *extraphysical precognitions* of the practitioner.

PENTA IS AN INEVITABLY DAILY PRACTICE.

Time. *Penta* has no relationship to a weekly rhythm, being a daily practice. The anonymous *extraphysical assistance* provided through *penta* should be performed daily, for example, in a brief period of 50 minutes between 6:00 and 9:00 p.m. (the *time of human anguish*). *Penta* should be performed *daily* and not exclude weekends, which bring the *"Sunday blues"* to the individual in lack, when they find themselves outside of their daily routine and are obliged to face the unpleasantness and emptiness in their life, which is generally unproductive from an evolutionary point of view.

Fixed. The above times are given as a standard example. One's schedule of *penta* can be different from this, depending on the personal conveniences of the penta candidate, as long as they are followed rigorously, 50 minutes within the specified 3 hours, in a daily period of 24 hours. The practitioner chooses a 3-hour period and makes it a *time fixed* forever. Examples: from 5:00 to 8:00 a.m.; from 7:00 to 10:00 p.m.; from 5:00 to 8:00 p.m.; from 9:00 p.m. to midnight.

De-soma. It is important to consider that, according to statistics, 6:00 p.m. is a critical time, as this is when the greatest number of individuals pass through the first death – also known as deactivation of the *soma, final projection*, biological death or brain death.

Continuity. After it is initiated, the practice of *penta* should not be interrupted for the rest of one's *intraphysical life*, due to the initial *intrusions* that the practitioner will be subject to, these being more incisive in the first 6 months.

Demands. In the initial 6 months, all types *of extraphysical consciousnesses* who are ill and in lack of affection and *consciential energy* will get used to your *set hour* for their absorption of energy and will *demand their quota of energy* in order to satisfy their needs until they feel freed from it.

Fatigue. The personal discipline of the practitioner demands that s/he avoid the practice of *penta* when tired, as this is always inconvenient in all respects. When this happens, it is best to invert the time of the task to the beginning of the day, in the morning, early morning or after various periods of sleep, for example.

Summer. Daylight saving time should be followed normally by the *penta practitioner.* This time shift is positive for the practitioner for reasons of temperature. Changes in *time zone* due to travel should also be followed, obviously avoiding the ill effects of *jetlag.*

Visits. Expected and unexpected visits to the house or apartment of the practitioner should not serve as obstacles in the daily practice of *penta.* This is resolved through the intelligent administration of one's schedule and plans of everyday life, joining obligations and responsibilities of daily life with the fixed assistential penta exercises. Personal *availability,* without self-corruption, for great *undertakings* increases as a direct result of one's healthy *motivations.*

Commitment. Ideally, the penta candidate will undertake the execution of this task with all possible realism regarding the gravity of the multi-dimensional or transcendent endeavor at hand – the most *committing* task that one could propose.

Difficulty. The commitment being *for the rest of one's life* is the most serious and difficult aspect in the practice of *penta.*

Aware. In this case, be aware and certain that this undertaking is *for the rest of your intraphysical life* – or, at least, until a heart attack, stroke, or some other incapacitating psychophysical accident permanently renders impossible the use of your person, *soma* and *holosoma* (the 4 vehicles of consciousness, when considered as a whole) in the delivery of direct or indirect *interconsciential* energetic assistance.

Mini-piece. This is the true condition of an *intraphysical mini*-piece within a multi-dimensional, assistential *maxi*-mechanism, characteristic of the practice of *penta,* and which the practitioner needs to understand without any personal doubt before making his or herself available to initiate this task.

SELF-DISORGANIZATION MAKES THE HEALTHY EXECUTION OF PENTA IMPOSSIBLE.

Self-disorganization. Self-disorganization also makes the performance of a *consciential epicenter* and the development of a *extraphysical clinic* impossible. This inhibits one's capacity of becoming a *consciential epicenter*, an *existential completist*, acquiring an *existential moratorium* or reaching the state of being *completely and permanently without intrusion.*

Competence. In penta, the basic rule in favor of the good of all evolutionary colleagues is: *we should only put those who are competent up-to-bat.*

Beginnings. An *intraphysical consciousness begins* to liberate him or herself from the multi-existential cycle when s/he *begins* to give good *extraphysical* examples. Penta predisposes one to these 2 beginnings simultaneously.

Trinomial. There is a very evident *interconsciential assistential trinomial* which manifests itself in a crescendo – each component being dependent on the other:

1. Consolation. *Assistential consolation task.*
2. Clarification. *Assistential clarification task.*
3. *Penta. Penta* or personal, daily, assistential, energetic task.

Holothosene. A very young *intraphysical consciousness'* attempt to implant the daily practice of *penta*, without the foundation of a well-consolidated existence, due to (*holothosenic pressure*, the influence of society, one's own *consciential basement* (predominance weak traits; see glossary), lack of experience, and *belly-brain),* is equivalent to attempting to have a *music therapy session* in a battlefield. The individual will hear the music at the same time that mortars are flying past his or her ears, or *para-ears.*

Trips. During the inevitable trips of human life, the *penta practitioner* will perform the exercises at the established hour, wherever he or she is.

Executive phase. For the reasons mentioned thus far, we can understand why the majority of candidates for penta only make themselves available to perform this assistential practice from 36 years of age onward, or rather, in the *executive phase* of human life, soon after the *preparatory* or educational *phase* from 1 to 35 years of age, within the average period of 7 decades of human life.

Duo. An *evolutionary duo* can develop the practices of penta in the *same place*, and on the *same bed*, as long as it is *not* performed at the *same time* or together.

Impossibilities. Following are summarized 9 variables or, more appropriately, 9 real impossibilities for the healthy development of the practice of *penta:*

1. *Intrusion.* Practitioner in the condition of being a victim of chronic *interconsciential intrusion.*

2. Self-corruption. Self-corruption on the part of the practitioner – man or woman.

3. Divorce. Divorce of the practitioner from his or her *Helper.*

4. Stagnation. Stagnation of the *consciousness* of the unmotivated practitioner, a practice of *stubbornness* or bad habits.

5. Idolatries. Cultivation of idolatries and establishment of sectarianisms on the part of the *penta practitioner* – a position based in the *belly-brain.*

6. Intention. The act of *thinking badly* of others, or having bad intentions, on the part of the practitioner – a grossly *anti-cosmoethical* condition.

7. *Soma.* The soma of the practitioner being seriously ill, or in a debilitated condition.

HUMAN WITNESSES ARE NOT PERMITTED DURING THE PRACTICE OF PENTA.

8. Witness. The practitioner allowing any human witness to be present in the room where he or she performs penta, while the task is in progress.

9. Go back. The practitioner wishing to go back on his or her assistential resolutions after initiating the practices. In order to develop, penta must be initiated with intelligence, in a definitive manner, without the possibility of any self-corrupting agreements or spurious pacts, from the very first moment, in the manner of *a path of abnegation with no return* or a liberating undertaking with no turning back.

7. ANTICIPATION OF PENTA

Anticipation. The following 3 technical conditions are more propitious to the useful anticipation of the experiences or practice of *penta:*

1. *Existential inversion.* *Existential inversion* by interested male or female youths is the best known process, at this time, that permits one to anticipate the practice of *penta* during the *preparatory phase* of one's *existential program* (up until 35 years of physical age) before the *executive phase* (on the average from 36 years of age on). Interested individuals should address themselves to the groups of *existential inverters.*

2. Itinerancy. The experience of itinerancy of the collaborator, or teacher of the International Institute of Projectiology (traveling to collaborate with the work of or to administer the seminar programs of IIPC internationally), can serve as a prologue, preparation, or first stage in the practice of *penta.*

3. *Existential recycling.* In certain cases, *existential recycling* (reprioritization to execute one's *existential program*), when precocious and at a high level, can also serve as an anticipation of the practices of *penta.* The interested individual, in this case, should seek out the group of *existential recyclers.*

8. DAILY CONTACTS

Abnegation. The first step of abnegation on the part of the *penta* practitioner is to initiate the daily energetic task with the liberation of *consciential energy* of the most benign, tranquil, conscious type possible, in favor of all those who s/he did not understand, *did not treat well*, or whom s/he misunderstood in an anti-fraternal manner during the last 24 hours.

Contacts. This provision – one of the most evolved of the *penta practitioner* – consists in calling up from your memory the images of the *intraphysical and extraphysical consciousnesses* from all *interconsciential* contacts during the day, mentalizing that a shower of energy is involving *consciousness*, with the sincere intention to place them in a *state of grace*, in the best condition possible, before your eyes.

The 4 following very characteristic types should be considered:

1. Direct physical contacts: greetings, encounters, conversations, visits, interviews, passengers, and others.
2. Indirect electro-electronic contacts: telephone, intercom, fax, fax/modem, and others.
3. Indirect mental contacts: letters, telegrams, conscious and unconscious evocations, reminiscences, and others.
4. Direct *extraphysical* contacts: *extraphysical* encounters through *lucid projections*, and others.

Signatures. This provision of *sanitation of the emotions* regarding one's daily contacts constitutes the cleansing of *dirty thosenic signatures*, left unresolved by the practitioner where s/he has been during the last 24 hours.

Good humor. This sanitation predisposes the personal condition of good humor in the practitioner from the beginning of every day.

9. EXPERIENCE

PENTA IS THE MAXIMAL EX-PERIENCE OF EVERYTHING THAT IS HEALTHY FOR CONSCIOUSNESSES.

Experience. Penta is a permanent *wholesale exercise* of everything that a *consciousness* knows, or specifically of the following 7 factors:

1. Discernment. Allows the practitioner to discerningly achieve the execution of his or her *existential project, completism*, and even *existential maxi-moratorium*.

2. *Holochakra*. Offers the *human consciousness* the means by which to install a more dense and permanent energetic field, or a subtle or densified *mist* beyond the aura, perceivable by any person disposed to do so, over men, women and children, in the most diverse human circumstances.

3. *Holomaturity*. Promotes the attainment of integrated maturity, beyond biological and psychological maturity.

4. *Mentalsomatics*. Facilitates the practitioner's employment of *consciential* attributes and individual potentials at a high level, and more than one personal intelligence at a time (we all have various types of intelligence).

5. *Multi-dimensionality*. Conducive of the *intraphysical consciousness'* inevitable attainment of the state of being *completely and permanently without intrusion*.

6. Psychic capacity. Permits the interested individual to accomplish *lucid pangraphy* (automatic writing).

7. Practicality. Indicates the means and recourses for the most rational experiential execution of human acts and *extraphysical* manifestations related to intraphysical life, in order for the *intraphysical consciousness* to be able to take advantage of the *consciential* dynamic in terms of his or her more lucid evolution.

10. SENSATIONS IN PENTA

Sensations. Upon the unmistakable action of an *extra-physical consciousness* over the vehicles of manifestation – in this case, the *soma* (human body), *holochakra* (energetic body), and *psychosoma* (emotional body) – of the *penta practitioner*, at least 33 unmistakable personal experiences can occur in the initial period of the *novice practitioner* of penta, when s/he *energetically and multi-dimensionally "stirs up the dust"* around him or herself, loved ones and things (men, women, children, subhumans, plants and *extraphysical consciousnesses* at various stages of evolution). Following are some of these sensations:

1. Asynchronization. The interference of ephemeral asynchronization between sounds and energetic transmissions are due to the difficulty of the *benign semi-possession*, or the coupling between the mind of the *intraphysical practitioner* and the *extraphysical Helper* who is responsible for the transmissions. The *Helper-possessor* commands, for example, one arm and the *possessed practitioner* commands the other.

2. Synchronization. The sounds of rhythmic vibrations heard inside the head during energetic discharges, are synchronous with the energetic "spraying" movements made with the arms and hands.

IMPROVEMENT OF THE ENERGETIC TRANSMISSIONS OF PENTA IS INCESSANT.

3. *Chakras.* After many years of these regular exercises, which are not regarded as a sacrifice, but are daily anticipated with sincere inner joy, the practitioner will perceive 4 of the major chakras simultaneously, while in the ordinary waking state:

A. *Sex-chakra.* The *sex-chakra* (primary or root chakra) pulses as though the practitioner were seated on a ball of fire. This is the so-called liberation of *kundalini,* which is greatly studied in Eastern Philosophy. In this case, its occurrence is definitively healthy or benign.

B. *Umbilical-chakra.* The *umbilical-chakra* (navel chakra) or the entire abdomen is energized towards the front. Not rarely, the abdomen appears to become thin and deformed like a fine sheet of paper.

C. *Frontal-chakra.* The *frontal-chakra* (third eye) appears to be a small, but powerful, apparatus encrusted in the forehead, functioning and perceiving outwards to a certain distance.

D. *Coronal-chakra.* The *coronal-chakra* (crown chakra) promotes an impressive sensation of the dissolving of one's own head.

4. Flame. Not rarely, the exteriorizations of *consciential energy* can give the impression that the *soma* (human body) becomes an enormous 10-foot-tall flame that is extremely hot on the outside and frozen at the center. This flame seems to crackle forward and upward, reverberating as though it were a center of light, expanding and contracting in alternately outward and inward movements, under the command of a controlled, intelligent, powerful and intangible force.

5. Flame-thrower. During the *benign semi-possession,* the *holochakra,* which is vitalizing the arms and hands to a greater degree, acts like a type of flame-thrower that is violently sending energy forward with discharges of a rapid and constant rhythm. The entire process is similar to the workings of an inter-dimensional-energetic-consciential-centrifuge.

THE HANDS OF THE PENTA PRACTITIONER CAN APPEAR TO BE ENERGETIC OUTLETS.

6. Clairvoyance. Diverse clairvoyant phenomena in the immediate area of the practitioner, or even remote viewing, with a high degree of lucidity.

7. Dematerialization. Sensation of dematerialization of fingers and hands.

8. Engage. The first energetic discharge serves more to *engage the psychic coupling* between the practitioner and the *extraphysical* transmitter. It is to be received by the therapeutic team, rather than being a *donation* for a *recipient consciousness (extraphysical consciousness* or projected individual).

9. Experiences. Obviously, the accumulation of daily experiences with penta will improve the performance of the dedicated practitioner and, with time, the *Helpers* will bring more greatly perturbed, ill *extraphysical consciousnesses* in order to approach the practitioner directly while in the waking state or even when s/he is projected with lucidity, outside of the scheduled time for *penta.* S/he will serve, in this case, as *assistential bait* (a condition wherein the individual is coupled with an ill *extraphysical consciousness* for therapeutic purposes), *aware* of his or her situation, both *intraphysically* and *extraphysically.* At this point, the *intraphysical-extraphysical rapport* intensifies, and the results of the energetic transmissions improve to unimaginable levels.

10. Extras. When the *penta practitioner* achieves an ability to work more closely with the *principal,* more permanent *extraphysical Helper* in the transmission of energies, extra or emergency energetic exteriorizations can occur, or rather: before (principally), during, or after the *penta* session. This can occur at unexpected moments or circumstances. When this happens, it is not in a physically or psychologically forced manner, but in one that is healthy, enriching and agreeable – without harmful or intrusive connotations. This is done in order to attend to the needs of ill *extraphysical consciousnesses* in a critical or emergency situation.

11. Phenomena. The healthy phenomena of *balloonment* (sensation of expansion) and *self-microscopy* (microscopic self-examination) are promoted by the expansion of the *holochakra.*

International Institute of Projectiology and Conscientiology (IIPC)

IIPC is a Brazilian, private, non-profit institution of research and education that studies *the consciousness*, placing special emphasis on the *out-of-body experience* (OBE). *Bioenergy*, an important factor in the occurrence of OBEs, and other altered states of consciousness, is also investigated.

The Institute holds educational lectures, seminars, conferences, workshops and courses at its 60 national and 8 international laboratory-schools in Barcelona, Buenos Aires, Caracas, Lisbon, London, Manhattan, Miami and Ottawa. Well over 20,000 individuals have taken IIPC courses.

IIPC offers its *Consciousness Development Program* (CDP), consisting of systematic experiential training in developing and controlling one's capacity to work with *bioenergy* and *out-of-body experience* (OBE).

To find out about other IIPC books and events contact the NY office at:

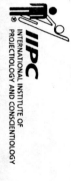

IIPC
INTERNATIONAL INSTITUTE OF
PROJECTIOLOGY AND CONSCIENTIOLOGY

2O East 49 Street, Suite 2F, New York, NY 10017
Tel./Fax: (718) 721-6257   E-mail: iipcnyusa@aol.com
http://members.aol.com/iipnyusa/iipc.htm

12. Cold. A sensation of cold air can affect the hands or the entire body. It can even chill the room of the practitioner, regardless of the ambient temperature.

13. *Holochakra.* During the energetic transmissions, the *soma* can sometimes appear smaller, or of a reduced volume. This is due to the expansion of the exteriorized *holochakra* (*mega-balloonment*).

14. Intensity. The *more intense* the energetic transmissions are, the *greater* will be the practitioner's *well-being* in the minutes or hours following the transmissions (post-*penta* period).

15. Intervals. The brief interval of time between one energetic transmission and another serves to physiologically replenish the practitioner and readjust the coupling between the practitioner and *Helper*, as well as to allow the substitution of the transmission-receiving *consciousness* (who may be close-by or far away) when necessary. The *Helper* generally does not lose energetic-mental-psychic control during this period. The intense sensations experienced by the practitioner can disappear during the intervals between 1 energetic discharge and another, maintaining him or her in a semi-possessed condition during the transmissions and somewhat free in the intervals.

16. Images. At this point, forceful images arise that are inspired by the *Helpers*, such as the following 3:

A. Galaxy. The incandescent creation of a solar system.

B. Furnace. The *flow of molten metal* inside the furnace of a steel plant.

C. Volcano. A sea of molten lava in an erupting volcano.

17. Machine. Frequently, during the energetic transmissions, the practitioner appears to hear the pulsing of an immense machine, as though all of his or her vehicles (*holosoma*), were coupled to an invisible and extremely powerful dynamo, serving as an intermediary part *(passe-partout)* of an unknown *extraphysical* machine.

18. Eighth. In general, one energetic discharge in 11 – the eighth, for example – can be perceivably more intense or potent than the others, due to the assistential work in progress.

THE TRANSMISSIONS ARE MADE WITH GENERALLY INTERMITTENT WAVES OF CONSCIENTIAL ENERGY.

19. Waves. In the practice of *penta,* transmissions are made with a specific type of wave of energy, which is generally perceived by the practitioner as being intermittent, and not continuous. Continuous waves of energy, when they do occur, imply a critical therapeutic circumstance, or a singular de-intrusive demand. These tend to be ephemeral, like an extraordinary or sporadic peak in the exteriorization of assistential energy.

20. *Projections.* The most diverse types of practical, lucid, *consciential projections* that are useful for both those assisted and the practitioner.

21. Itching. One of the first indications of physical effect phenomena, or the exteriorization of ectoplasm, is a non-habitual itching in the nasal passages, during penta. This is due to the excretion of ectoplasm through the mucous membranes of the human body's orifices.

22. Psychophony. Psychophonic monologue is the phenomenon wherein an *extraphysical consciousness* (in this case, the *Helper*) uses the *projector's soma* to speak directly to the body's owner (the practitioner during *penta*) who is temporarily projected. As you can see, psychophonic monologue is a rare, transcendent inversion of conditions, positions of *consciousnesses* and *interconsciential* manifestations.

23. Pulsations. Energy pulsations in the brain. It is important to note that the brain, physiologically speaking, does not pulse, per se, as the heart does, for example. In this case, the bizarre sensations felt are actually those of *pulsations* occurring inside the head. Regarding these sensations and the majority of references made here, the individual will only be able to better evaluate his or her own details and healthy effects with the pas-

sage of time and the expansion of his or her development in assistential practices.

24. Quality. Time does not represent a relevant factor in the energetic discharges. What is much more important is the quality and the potentiality (potential, capacity) of the *consciential energies* transmitted.

25. Rhythm. Not rarely, the varied and intense rhythm of the energetic discharges, physical movements and muscular contractions, practically does not alter the *heart rate* of the practitioner. This fact alone constitutes a separate, concomitant, subjective phenomenon.

26. *Independence.* Strictly speaking, the always perceivable frequency of the energetic transmissions of the practitioner are not affected by the following variables:

A. Will. Neither the practitioner's *will* nor his or her intention.

B. Circulation. Your *heart beats*, which maintain blood circulation, being the most demanding and important area, concerning the cerebral hemispheres.

C. Respiration. Your *respiratory frequency* that maintains your *oxygen supply* and is directly connected with the *cardiochakra.*

D. Time. The ticking of *seconds* that measures human chronological time.

27. Orders. Everything happens under the supervisory psychic command of the principle *extraphysical* transmitter. Nevertheless, the transmission set seems to be coupled to powerful *extraphysical* apparatuses that are still unknown at this stage of our leading-edge understanding. Four or five different rhythms of *energetic transmissions* that differ greatly from one another can occur in a singular assistential session of 10 basic transmissions.

28. *Soma.* Movements in the position of the soma which is laying down on the bed.

29. Sounds. The sounds of the vibrations generated by the energy passing through the head of the penta practitioner, can appear to pass through the arms and hands. In this case, it can

seem as though tambourines are being beaten with intelligence, or the repeating cadence of a *mantra* – a singular word that is not pronounced, but repeatedly heard, with greater or lesser acceleration.

30. Numbness. A lack of feeling, especially in the face and lips.

31. Transmitters. The *extraphysical*, energetic transmitters, or *Helpers,* can trade-off among themselves during a singular session. The aware *intraphysical*-practitioner-*projector* will perceive the alternation and technical changes that are characteristically individual and unmistakable. The man or woman's *para-sensation* is, not rarely, quite unique.

32. Experiences. Many *non-specific sensations* and physical and *psychic experiences* can occur in a constant crescendo, with limits that are undefined or unknown at the present time, by all of us, during the practice of *penta.*

PSYCHIC PHENOMENA CAN OCCUR SIMULTANEOUSLY WITH PENTA.

33. Simultaneous. The 2 following examples are worth noting as psychic phenomena that can appear simultaneously with *penta:*

A. Tachycardia. The intensive and extreme physical movement of the arms without the appearance of tachycardia (elevated heart rate) or increased levels of adrenaline in the circulatory system. This fact is still obscure and apparently antiphysiological (paradoxical).

B. Digestion. The unexpected acceleration of digestion in certain circumstances of emergency assistance.

11. SEXUAL CONNECTIONS

Energetics. It is best that the practitioner not forget 4 realities regarding *consciential energy:*

1. **Life.** Life, in any dimension, is assistance between *consciousnesses.*

2. **Assistentiality.** Assistance between *consciousnesses* is that which signifies energetics, *bio*energetics and *para*energetics.

3. **Embryology.** Life is energetic, and has its beginning on Earth with embryology or through the sexual act (energy and adrenaline).

4. **Predominance.** Human life is, after all, predominately *holochakral* (energetic).

Holochakra. The *holochakra* is the *energetic para-body* of *consciential energies* of each man and woman. The *holochakra* is the *para-body* of *pre-kundalini*, of *kundalini*, of the *sex-chakra (sex-soma)*, as well as all dense physical energies.

Connections. The holochakra has 2 connections.

1. **Mini-connection.** The *mini*-connection in the *soma* or human body.

2. **Maxi-connection.** The more important *maxi*-connection in the *psychosoma.*

Trinomial. The 2 connections of the *holochakra* constitute the trinomial *soma-holochakra-psychosoma*, within the *holosoma* or the set of vehicles of manifestation of *human consciousness.*

De-soma (death). The rupture of the holochakra's mini-connection causes *de-soma,* or the biological death of the *soma.*

Sex-soma. The integral human personality is the one who is *sexually active,* with the identification, acceptance and experience of a basic sexual instinct.

THE SEXUALLY INACTIVE HUMAN CONSCIOUSNESS IS AN ENERGETICALLY DEFICIENT PERSONALITY.

Deficiency. The *sexually inactive intraphysical consciousness* can be seen as an *energetically deficient* human personality.

Sex. Without the *active* maxi-connection of your *holochakra* with the *psychosoma,* promoted by daily sex, an *intraphysical consciousness* becomes *sexually inactive.* In this case, he or she is not able to fluently develop *penta.* Only the practice of daily sex allows one to maintain the *active* maxi-connection of the *sexually active intraphysical consciousness.* Penta with the mature sexuality of the practice of daily sex is a developing *penta,* independent of the gender or physical age of the practitioner.

Influx. *Consciential energy* flows more intensely from the *psychosoma* to the *soma* between 1 and 35 years of age, for the individual having an average life span of 7 decades. This can be considered the *influx* of energy or the vitalizing *entrance* of the *consciousness' energy* in *intraphysical life.*

Outflow. *Consciential energy* flows more intensely from the *soma* to the *psychosoma* between 35 and 70 years of physical age. This can be considered the *outflow* of energy or the *return* of *consciousness* to its real, *extraphysical precedence.*

PENTA WITHOUT DAILY SEX ON THE PART OF THE PRACTITIONER ONLY ACHIEVES HALF-STRENGTH.

Half-strength. *Penta without daily sex* is a stationary *penta* that only achieves half-strength, because this condition makes it more difficult to achieve a more expressive evolutionary *consciential* growth.

Warnings. The following 5 procedures are not recommended in the practice of *penta*:

1. Companion. A woman *without a companion* is not even able to give assistance to the one she loves. How, then, can she perform assistance to other *intraphysical* and *extraphysical consciousnesses?* The woman *with companionship* begins her assistentiality in a healthy or energetically shielded bedroom. This is a condition that is completely different and much more effective in the development of *penta.* The same occurs with the man who *has* or *does not have* companionship.

2. Masturbation. Masturbation is an *atypical behavior* that should not be employed as a typical behavior for the rest of one's *intraphysical life.* This is because it does not satisfy the need for sexual alleviation with personal energies or the calming the sexual hyper-excitability naturally generated through the practice of *penta.*

3. Sublimation. Any useless attempt at sublimation of sex, for whatever reason, is castration, or physical *somatic* energetic human mutilation. This is one more condition that makes the maintenance of the practice of *penta,* with a mature, secure and healthy development quite impractical.

4. Menopause. Menopause must not turn a *woman* into a *eunuch* for the remainder of the exercises practiced in *penta.* In order to avoid this, modern medicine knows how to effectively deal with menopause through the balancing of hormones and the indication of an active sex life.

5. Old age. Old age, or the stage of life's veterans, after 65 years, should not turn a man or a woman into a *sexual vege-*

table. This is another condition that does not function with penta, with which energetic life is more intense, long-lasting or as permanent as possible.

Relief. Healthy *congressus subtilis* (sexual relationships between physical and *extraphysical consciousnesses*) between a practitioner and a *Helper* can occur, upon the initiative of the assistential maxi-mechanism, in order to alleviate the individual in a period of travel, separation or when widowed – in a temporary fashion.

Jealousy. An evolutionary duo (two individuals working together in an evolutionary synergistic manner) must seriously observe the processes of jealousy, possessiveness and affectionate or psychological insecurity relative to the assistance practiced through penta. For example, if a woman becomes jealous because of telephone calls from other women who are requesting assistance from the male practitioner (her mate) through the practice of *penta,* she will join forces entirely and *position herself shoulder-to-shoulder with the intruders.* These *intruders* are not only those of *consciousness* that is to be treated, but of the individuals who telephoned soliciting help, those of the practitioner, and the jealous woman's as well. The practitioner, in this case, will be cornered and will feel this directly and immediately with his *para-senses.* It is easy to imagine what can arise in the way pathology in this atmosphere of misunderstanding between the partners of an evolutionary duo. In the same manner, a male can become jealous of the requests for assistance being made to his female partner.

Intercourse. Sexual relations *shortly before* the practice of penta are not recommended due to assistential preparations on the part of the Helpers. After practicing penta, sexual relations do not present any logical inconvenience.

12. ASSISTENTIAL OPERATIONS

Operations. The spasmodic, frenetic, synchronous spreading movements made with the arms and hands during the energetic transmissions, are intended to assist *intraphysical* and *extraphysical consciousnesses* through the 3 following distinct and generally interconnected operations:

1. Donation. Exteriorization of *immanent energy* and *consciential energy*.
2. Dematerialization. Transitory dematerialization of *parts* of the practitioner's *soma*.
3. Ectoplasmy. Extraction of dense, human energy, or *ectoplasm*, exclusively for therapeutic, or, more appropriately, *para-therapeutic* purposes.

Outlets. The *para*-arms and *para*-hands of the penta practitioner's *psychosoma* serve as energetic outlets or spreaders, under the unmistakable, perceivable and real command of the *Helper* – the real transmitter of *consciential energy*.

Musculature. Those who practice *penta,* giving psychic passivity to the assistential technicians, end up with more muscular arms, shoulders and thorax. The pectoral muscles also become more voluminous and rigid, thus increasing one's muscular mass and, consequently, body mass, due to the daily physical exercises.

AN AMBIENT TEMPERATURE BELOW 68°F FACILITATES THE PRACTICE OF PENTA.

Temperature. An ambient temperature below 68°F predisposes an intensification of the exteriorization of consciential energies.

Observations. In order to maintain affinity, cohesion, attunement, balance, and intensify operation during the vibrational state (VS) that occurs during the greater exteriorizations of *consciential energy*, the *Helper* makes observations or gives opportune psychic suggestions, which are generally irresistible on the part of the *penta practitioner.*

Reflections. Among the psychic suggestions made by the *Helper*, one of them will lead the *penta practitioner*, when more conscious, to inevitably reflect upon *concepts* that at first seem disparate, but are related to each other and the assistential service at hand with unquestionably logical connections.

Consciousnesses. *Penta* develops through 3 interconnected *consciousnesses:*

1. Practitioner. The *intraphysical penta practitioner* (adult man or woman).
2. *Helper.* An *extraphysical Helper(s)* having the appearance of a man or a woman. He or she can occasionally be a *super-Helper* or a *karmic group's evolutionary orientor.*
3. Assisted. Those *extraphysical* or *intraphysical consciousnesses* who are being *assisted.*

Encapsulation. *Para-sanitary encapsulation* is assistential isolation and temporary, energetic annulment of the manifestations of one's *thosenes* (thoughts, sentiments or emotions and energy) – notably the intrusive thosenes of one or more ill *intraphysical* or *extraphysical consciousness.* This operates in the same way that sanitary isolation (quarantine) exists in hospitals with inpatients having infectious or contagious diseases who present a high capacity for toxic, radioactive or disease contamination.

EXTRAPHYSICAL SANITARY ENCAPSULATION IS A COMMON OCCURRENCE WITH THE PENTA PRACTITIONER.

Perception. The occurrence of *extraphysical* sanitary encapsulation is not always clearly perceived by the *penta practi-*

tioner. This is because the isolation is sponsored by one or, more frequently, several *Helpers* working together, and, not rarely, transcends your perceptive capacity.

Classification. *Extraphysical* sanitary encapsulation can be classified into 3 types in terms of *consciousnesses,* time and *consciential* dimensions:

1. *Consciousnesses.* Encapsulation of *intraphysical* and *extraphysical consciousnesses* can be individual, conjugal (duo), or collective (group).

2. Time. Encapsulation can last for minutes, hours or days.

3. Dimensions. In terms of space or *consciential* dimensions, the isolation can include *intraphysical* and *extraphysical consciousnesses* of a home or apartment, an entire apartment building, or even a neighborhood or metropolis.

Philosophy. The philosophy of the anti-entropical, *interconsciential* assistentiality of *para-sanitary* encapsulation is based on the practical premise that *not getting in the way is already very helpful.*

Urban renewal. *Extraphysical* sanitary isolation is an extraordinary aid in the services of *extraphysical urban renewal* – changes for the better in pathological *extraphysical* ambiances and communities. It is sponsored by the *serenissimus* (a consciousness that is soon to pass through the third death).

Gratification. It is gratifying and always comforting for the *penta practitioner* to be aware of his or her participation in cases of para-sanitary isolation and *extraphysical urban renewal,* even if it is but a *small contribution* to the effective assistential work of the *Invisible College of Serenissimus.*

13. HELPERS

Elementary. The elementary *penta practitioner* is the man or woman who does not evolve or progress to more developed *Helpers.*

THE HELPER IS THE EXTRAPHY-SICAL CO-PRACTITIONER IN THE PERFORMANCE OF PENTA.

Maintenance. The elementary *penta practitioner* always has a *Helper* only for the maintenance of his or her sub-level assistential tasks in comparison with his or her real multi-dimensional, energetic, psychic possibilities that have not yet been taken advantage of. This condition exists because the practitioner does not allow him or herself to improve, due to repressions, physical and mental laziness, neophobia and other weak traits, or fissures in their personality.

Supervision. The *Helper* that supervises the multi-dimensional assistential work of the *extraphysical clinic,* together with the *consciential epicenter (penta practitioner),* is different from the *Helper* that supervises the *benign semi-possession* of *penta.*

Communication. It is imperative that the practitioner communicate with the *Helper.* This is an indispensable measure in *penta.*

Passivity. The practitioner who *remains silent* during the practice of *penta, communicates* with the *Helper* by remaining psychically passive and receptive.

Intimacy. *Communication is cohabitation.* Your intimacy with the *Helper* is greater than the intimacy with one's *partner* in the condition of conventional marriage or *partnership* in an *evolutionary duo.* This is due to the *holosomatic coupling* between the *penta practitioner* and the *Helper.*

Partnerships. There are 2 very different types of partnerships in terms of *interconsciential* intimacies:

1. Simple. The *simpler* partnership in an *evolutionary duo*, or in a conventional marriage, which is basically formed through the *soma*.

2. Complex. The *more complex* partnership between the *penta practitioner* and the *Helper*, which is basically formed through the *holosoma*.

Potentiality. Thus, the energy of the veteran *penta practitioner* consistently increases in its potentiality (potential, capacity), through the actions of the *Helper* who works through the *holosoma*.

Wisdom. The wisdom of the *Helpers* is shown in the just *cosmoethical* dosage used in everything they do. They never *leave out* what is necessary and never *let things go too far*, regardless of whether the issue is *interconsciential* assistance, the use of *consciential energy*, or the employment of the practitioner's talents in the role of a sensitive assistential instrument.

14. MENTALSOMATICITY

Concepts. Following are 13 examples of *complex ideas (Mentalsomaticity,* the *tho* of *thosene)* that will come to the mind of the penta practitioner according to his or her more frequent *intellectual motivations,* archetypes, and the quality and extent of his or her *cerebral dictionary.*

1. Self-conduct. The self-sufficiency of *intraphysical consciousness.*

2. Black hole. A black hole is the state that matter reaches after suffering a gravitational collapse from which no light, material or any other type of signal can escape.

3. *Uncreated creator.* The so-called *First Cause.*

4. The "n"th power.

5. Eternity. Here, eternity signifies life that seems, to us, to continue forever in a cycle of rebirths and deaths.

6. Phoenix. The myth of the rebirth of the phoenix.

7. Implosion. The condition of *oneness; consciousness* in a state of being one with the universe.

8. The infinity of the future. What happens after the condition of free *consciousness* (the state of *consciousness* after discarding the *psychosoma* at the end of the rebirth cycle)?

9. The infinity of the past. The beginning of everything.

10. Perpetual motion. A continuous physical motor, being a caricature of a mechanical steel wheel, without electricity or any other resource, that gyrates incessantly, powered only by gravity.

11. Omnipotence. Omnipotence is absolute authority or rule.

12. *Bottomless pit.* Abyss; maelstrom; *void.*

13. Information highway. The information superhighway, here, signifies the maximum current vanguard of practical *intraphysical* universalism.

15. HOLOCHAKRALITY

Development. As a *consciousness* becomes more evolved, s/he will have a more intense energetic potential, and will require less *consciential* effort and time to complete its *energetic recuperation* (*sympathetic assimilations and deassimilations*).

Consciential energy. *Consciential energy* is inexhaustible.

Mobilization. The factor that generates the development of the *intraphysical* practitioner's psychic abilities is the sensed, voluntary, conscious fluency with his or her energies. For this reason, the more developed *intraphysical* being – from a psychic, animic, and energetic point of view – will always be the one that presents a mastery of mobilization, exteriorization, absorption and maintenance of the self-defensive circulation of energies; a looseness of the *holochakra*; the projection of the psychosoma; the efficient recall of *extraphysical* events; and other developments of an equal nature.

Re-education. One does not develop only a single type of psychic ability or only one determinate animic phenomenon. What one intrinsically develops in one's *consciential* microuniverse is the *conscious mobilization of energy*, which generates and unleashes all psychic phenomena. This development is a re-education for each *new* human existence, *new holochakra* and *new soma*.

Duration. In the *beginning*, the energetic irradiations of the *penta* exercises can last up to 50 minutes or *1 hour*, within the 3-hour period chosen in the 24 hours of each day.

Discharges. With the daily development of the penta practices, and the maximal technical development of the practitioner, 11 discharges of *consciential energy* can be accomplished in only 25 to 45 minutes of an individual 1-hour session.

Contractions. Each energetic discharge corresponds to at least 50 transmission-contractions. Eleven discharges come to an average total of 550 transmissions by the end of each daily period.

IDEALLY, PENTA SHOULD BE EXECUTED FAR FROM MEAL TIMES.

Meals. It is necessary to observe the time and the quantity of food that the practitioner ingests a little before the daily exercises, in order to avoid the extra work of *digestive acceleration* on the part of the *Helpers*. After practicing *penta*, there is no problem with the practitioner eating, which occurs with a certain frequency due to the appetite provoked by the physical exercises.

Extraphysical clinic. In a more advanced state of the practice of *penta,* the *Helpers* transform the projector's *physical base* into a mobile *extraphysical medical clinic,* or rather, a *extraphysical clinic* that is dedicated to the assistance of *intraphysical* and *extraphysical consciousnesses* who are in lack.

Isolation. The *extraphysical clinic* is a type of quarantine area of an *extraphysical* hospital that is reserved to temporarily receive ill *extraphysical consciousnesses* inside of a transitional *interdimensional bubble.*

Periods. There are 2 very characteristic periods in the practice of *penta* (see chap. 10).

1. The *pre-penta* period, before the installation of the daily assistential services.

2. The *post-penta* period, after the daily realization of assistential services.

16. OBJECTS

Instruments. It is not recommended that you leave any type of instrument or apparatus turned on or functioning inside of the room where you practice *penta*, during the exercises. This is due to the physical effects of a psychic or ectoplasmic origin. For example: computer, telephone, intercom, TV, *beeper*, VCR with digital clock and lights, noisy clock, and others.

Firearms. The *energetically shielded bedroom*-laboratory, physical base, *projectarium*, or *extraphysical clinic* of the *penta practitioner, obviously, should not* be used to store arms of any nature – firearms, for example.

Contact lenses. The *penta practitioner* should develop his or her daily energetic-animic-psychic sessions without contact lenses on his or her eyes. Use of *extended wear* contact lenses *is not recommended* in the course of *penta* practices.

Prosthetics. The use of glasses, rings, earrings, watches and other objects that are temporarily removable – a false or prosthetic leg, for example – should be avoided during the practices of *penta.*

Menstruation. A woman's menstrual period does not necessarily affect her practice of *penta.* Quite the opposite; it can stabilize her hormonal system through her own energy.

IUD. *It is not recommended* that a woman use an IUD (intra-uterine device), a foreign object inside an organ as noble as the uterus of the *soma* and its *consciential energies*, in the development of the *penta* practice.

Drawer. Ideally, the veteran penta practitioner will keep a drawer reserved where he or she can keep only those *papers, letters, telegrams, faxes with requests for interconsciential assistance* at a distance which he or she will inevitably receive, upon his or her permanent assistential task becoming more well known.

Types. With the development of the assistential practice of *penta*, the practitioner can come to seem like a *company*, as he or she will receive solicitation from 4 diverse types of communication:

1. Mail: the practitioner receives letters or telegrams addressed to his or her *extraphysical clinic*, with requests for assistance at a distance.
2. Memos: internal communications from within a *conscientiological* company requesting assistance.
3. Fax: requests for assistance by fax.
4. Computers: solicitations for assistance via computer network.

Registration. One of the most serious facets required for the maintenance of correct conduct on the part of the practitioner is discretion regarding assistential facts and personalities that directly or indirectly participate, and about whom they give information. You should not register any phenomenological data that involves those who are assisted in the penta practices, in order to avoid *spurious evocations*.

Experiences. If the practitioner wishes to make note of his or her experiences, s/he should do so only in regards to personal sensations and developments in order to amplify understanding and efficient collaboration with the *Helpers*, and not involve him or herself with the pathologies or *para-pathologies* of others. S/he who seeks to help, needs to maintain him or herself in the best condition possible in order to be able to assist. This measure aids the *sympathetic de-assimilations* of energy.

Bedside lamp. It is advisable to maintain the habit of keeping a bedside lamp at the head of the bed – on the *night stand* – in order to facilitate the observation of your movements in the room where you practice penta, especially after the daily exercises.

Clock. When possible, it is best to keep a small digital clock next to the bedside lamp on the night stand in order to better control time and discipline yourself in regards to the development of *penta.*

THE USE OF AN ALARM CLOCK IS NOT RECOMMENDED IN THE PRACTICE OF PENTA.

Alarm clock. Ideally, one will make his or her own *biological clock* work in order to wake up at the exact time desired from the *penta* session. In this way, the practitioner will experience his or her *interconsciential* assistance with discretion. An alarm clock can serve, in many cases, to *convoke intruders* through the irritation it provokes (loud impact).

Notes. With the development of the assistential energetic exercises, the best idea is to always keep loose sheets of *white paper* for notations, as well as a fine blue felt-tip *pen*, in order to note the inspirational reflections and original ideas you receive soon after the penta exercises, and later enter them into your personal computer.

A PERMANENT PHYSICAL BASE IN A HOTEL IS NOT IDEAL FOR THE DAILY PRACTICE OF PENTA.

Hotel. Obviously, the *intraphysical consciousness* who lives in a hotel, has this apartment as a physical base. A hotel, used as a permanent, definitive, physical base *is not ideal* for the practices of *penta* due to the tumult of the locale, with people coming and going, generally in critical existential periods, right outside of your residence.

Paradoxes. Having a hotel as a physical base generates 3 points for reflection regarding the *paradoxes* of the *penta* practitioner's life:

1. Provisionality. S/he does not get attached to human life because he or she does not live with the sensation of the provisionality that the hotel resident-guest has.

2. Responsibility. S/he is very aware that s/he is in transit through *intraphysical* life. S/he does not fear physical death, but, nonetheless, maintains responsibility in terms of his or her human obligations.

　　　　3. *Existential program.* S/he is *bound to nothing*, just as the resident-guest is not, but feels *tied down to everything* in terms of the completion of his or her *existential program.*

　　　　Euphoria. One of the down-sides of the practice of *penta* is also one of its benefits: the production of euphoria in the practitioner. This euphoria needs to be controlled, without repression, in order to not compromise the passivity of the *penta practitioner.*

17. GROUP

Group. Penta does not work in a group setting as it is an individual commitment. The group nature in its practice is multidimensional, following the directives of an assistential maximechanism.

Practices. Following are 5 practices that are similar, as are many others, but are not identical to and do not produce the same results as *penta:*

1. Religious service held once a week in the home. This is common in the Brazilian spiritist movement.
2. *Mediumistic* session held in a group setting, in private or in public *(de-intrusion)*, once a week. This is performed in various *mediumistic* sects.
3. The whirling dances of Umbanda (a Brazilian spiritual practice, originating in Africa).
4. Transmission of Communion of Thought, in general held for 5 minutes at 6:00 p.m. daily, without any greatly fixed commitment.
5. Third part of the rosary (prayer) of the Catholic Church.

JUST AS HALF-PREGNANCY DOES NOT EXIST, NEITHER DOES HALF-PENTA EXIST.

Stationary. A stationary penta only achieves half-strength (see chap. 11), which is different from half-*penta.*

18. COUNTER-INDICATIONS OF PENTA

Counter-indications. It *is not recommended* that the following 6 types of individuals practice *penta:*

1. Ignorant. The one who *has never felt* ostensive, *intraconsciential, psychic manifestations,* and who refuses to discuss the subject, being uninformed regarding the theme, or who can be classified as *psychically ignorant.*

2. Beginner. Those who are initiates or beginners regarding psychic matters (bioenergy, animism and mediumship), who are still not developed to a reasonable, individual, practical level.

3. Mini-intrusion. Those victims of eventual unconscious *mini-intrusions,* or rather: the *great majority* of the planetary population. One who is already pathologically *super*-possessed by an *intruder,* cannot be benignly *semi*-possessed by a *Helper.* This fact confirms a principle of physics, physiology, *para-physiology* and *Conscientiology:* "two bodies cannot occupy the same space, at the same time, in the same dimension."

4. Uncontrolled. Those unrefined *intraphysical consciousnesses* who cannot control their psychic processes of *consciential* exchange (mediumship) in a healthy, comfortable manner. Those who, for example, suffer uncontrollable, incessant myoclonia (twitches) when they are near *extraphysical consciousnesses.*

THOSE WHO ARE AVID FOR TROPOSPHERIC (PHYSICAL) SENSATIONS ARE STILL NOT READY FOR PENTA.

5. Avid. Those *intraphysical consciousnesses* who are still anxious for instinctual sensations, who have not yet determined their human intentions and aspirations; in general, those of 35 physical years and under, who are in the *phase* of their life

that is *preparatory* to the execution of their *existential program*. He or she who wants to practice penta only when they have 2 million dollars in the bank is wasting their time, as they will never achieve good assistential results with *penta*.

6. Children. Obviously, the practice of *penta* is not recommended for children of either sex, at any infantile age, even if they are psychically gifted.

19. PENTA TEST

Test. Chapter 345 of the book *"700 Conscientiology Experiments"* is a test regarding penta. It has been reproduced below, in general terms, in order to offer more clarity on the subject.

Evolution. A *consciousness* only evolves more rapidly when he or she helps other *consciousnesses* to evolve. This summarizes the evolutionary dynamic that affects us all.

Conscientiotherapy. The daily practice of penta affects the inevitable inner renovation of the *intraphysical consciousness.* It is incompatible for the *penta practitioner* to maintain the following 30 habits or *anticosmoethical* behaviors:

1. Rely on divinations in your day-to-day decisions.

2. Knock on wood any number of times, being a slave to an irrational superstition.

3. Carry a rabbit's foot or sacred items around your neck or in your shirt.

4. Habitually cry once a week out of great insecurity and dissatisfaction.

5. Naively collect firearms; a fundamental imprudence.

6. Cultivate any kind of guru-worship or *consciential* self-subjection.

7. Cultivate a chronically pessimistic point of view regarding the universe.

8. Make irrational promises, or rather: not trust in multi-dimensionality (the multi-dimensional team).

9. Smoking: a primitive addiction and an irreparable blocker of the *cardio-chakra's consciential energy.*

10. Work as a professional animal killer.

11. Keep a shrine or altar in your home, under the yoke of infantile mysticism.

12. Maintain excessive body weight (psychological obesity), increased by bulimia or a sedentary life.

13. Spend entire nights promiscuously several nights a month (intrudability).

14. Think and worry only about your nuclear family *(mega-ego-karma).*

15. Practice *bird hunting,* for example, or the condition of pathological zoo-conviviality (interrelationship with animals).

16. Continue to live a disorganized life.

17. Feel manifest or transparent insecurity in your daily acts.

18. Be a motorcyclist, with the high energetic risk it involves.

19. Support, even sincerely, the death penalty.

20. Be a pathological user of alcohol or drugs in general, be they light or heavy ones.

21. Suffer habitual unconscious *mini-intrusions* that are evident to others.

22. Have and use arms, in a conscious evocation of sub-human killing.

23. Spend all your time unproductively, without any creativity.

24. Have an occupation that contributes, to any degree, towards the repression of *consciousnesses.*

25. Work *heavily* with a chain saw in any rural area (pathological fito-conviviality (interaction with plants).

26. Live in a state of permanent unsociability, or as a hermit in a convent.

27. Live tied to a sectarian doctrine, in mediocre, medieval anti-universalism.

28. Live with the depressive habit of taking *mood-altering drugs* or depressants.

29. Continuously live without a fixed intraphysical residence or in an impulsive nomadism.

30. Fly using a hang-glider: free flight is a high risk, lethal or suicidal sport.

Habits. If you still participate in even 3 of these personal habits, rest assured: you are *far from* being able to perform healthy, effective *penta.*

20. INDICATIONS OF PENTA

Indications. It is recommended that only the following 4 types of *intraphysical consciousness* perform the daily, scheduled practice of *penta:*

1. Veterans. *Intraphysical consciousnesses* who are more-or-less psychically developed or are veterans in terms of *energetic and psychic self-defense.*

ONE OF THE GOALS OF PENTA IS TO DEVELOP THE HUMAN CONSCIOUS-NESS TOWARDS THE CONDITION OF BEING COMPLETELY AND PERMA-NENTLY WITHOUT INTRUSION.

2. *De-intrusion.* Those *intraphysical consciousnesses* without *greater* problems of *intrusion,* entirely secure in what they are doing. It is not necessary that an *intraphysical consciousness* be or live completely and permanently without intrusion. Quite to the contrary, the *intraphysical consciousness* develops towards the state of being *completely and permanently without intrusion* through the performance of *penta,* with gradual, *consciential self-de-intrusion,* executed through the daily, *de-intrusion* of patients – ill *extraphysical* and *intraphysical consciousnesses* – who are at a distance. *Penta* is the ideal technique for *anti-intrusive self-defense* of a multi-dimensional nature.

3. Flexible. Lucid *intraphysical consciousnesses* having *holochakral* flexibility, capacity with the *vibrational state,* reception and absorption of *consciential energy,* and the dozens of existing bioenergetic techniques that are applicable and are exercised on a daily basis.

4. Prisoners. *Penta,* as is *lucid consciousness projection,* is especially indicated for practice by prisoners who generally wish to improve the direction of their personal destiny but are

incapacitated, finding themselves physically removed from their fellow human beings – as long as they fit within the outlined parameters and have the *strong* traits outlined previously. Due to his or her circumstances, the penta of a prisoner will only achieve half-strength, in view of the characteristics of their affective and sex life, and other repressions.

Mega-challenge. *There are more counter-indications* than indications in the daily practice of *penta*. This is because the daily *personal energetic task* is the greatest assistential, psychic, energetic challenge that 1 *intraphysical consciousness* can undertake – for *the rest of their intraphysical existence* – in our current intraphysical society, which is still pathological, according to leading-edge *Conscientiology* research.

Extraphysical clinic. Penta is the ideal resource for the maintenance of balance and energetic homogeneity of the *intraphysical consciousness' extraphysical clinic.*

Self-sacrifice. The daily *personal energetic task* is a practice that sometimes demands sacrifices, but it is an unparalleled resource for the evolutionary dynamization of the practitioner and his or her loved ones.

Restoration. The assistential-psychic-energetic exercises of *penta* always energetically restore the practitioner, in his or her contact with the *extraphysical* assistants in their *pacific intrusions* or *healthy semi-possessions*, and the temporary experience in other *consciential* dimensions.

21. APPLICATIONS OF PENTA

Application. *Penta* is the best application of an individual's energy.

Applications. There are innumerous evolutionary, *holokarmic* applications for penta; among them, the following 7:

1. Protection. Penta maintains a positive *extraphysical* protection, a *protective shell*, or *good*, permanent, multidimensional *assistance*, for the human life of the *projector*, as well as the achievement of *super-health*.

2. *Continuous*. The habit of exteriorizing assistential energies can promote a more structured ego in the practitioner, yielding the most elevated state of balance that an *intraphysical consciousness* can attain. At this point your *mentalsoma* will almost always become coupled with the *mentalsoma* of 1 aware *consciousness* or an *evolutionary orientor*, in the serene and evolved state of *continuous consciousness*.

3. *Hyper-thosenes*. The state or period of time of the energetic transmissions during the practice of *penta*, shows itself to be highly propitious for the assimilation of new ideas, or *hyper-thosenes* on the part of the attentive practitioner.

4. *Parapathology*. One of the basic applications of *penta* is the sanitization of *parapathological* disturbances of the *psychosoma*. Among these is the consequence of intraphysical restriction suffered by the *extraphysical consciousness* who recently passed through de-soma. For example: the quicker recuperation of *extraphysical* maturity for those *consciousnesses* who suffered physical death at a physically tender age or during adolescence and become *extraphysical* children who deserve or need to return to a status of *consciential* adulthood as quickly as possible. In these cases, the dense tropospheric energy of the *penta practitioner* acts in a positive manner with the possibility of having a greater *rapport* in the extraction of energies that are still very human and connected to the *extraphysical consciousness*.

5. *Energetic spring*. Penta allows the practitioner to calibrate the energetic condition of his or her day, week, or the

current period of his or her human existence, including the evolutionary periods of *energetic spring* (period of abundant healthy energy).

6. Recesses. The assistential exteriorization of *consciential energy* with a fixed, pre-scheduled time that is maintained with discipline and perseverance, is the best technique for the veteran conscious *projector* to avoid prolonged recess in the agile production of *conscious projections*. On the other hand, one can overcome recesses in the intensity and quality of assistential services performed in penta that are similar to those which occur in one's *conscious projections*.

7. *Existential program*. The regular execution of assistance to other imbalanced *consciousnesses* with *penta*, inevitably makes you observe the use of your *holosoma* and the maintenance of your own *soma* with greater attention and care – as well as everything that has to do with your hygiene, health, use of personal bioenergy, self-discipline, and the increasing realization of obligations pertaining to your *existential program*.

Dimensions. *Consciential energies* act beyond space and time. There are various dimensions that are closer to our *thosenic* manifestations. Among those that pertain to the practice of *penta*, we can point out the following 3. They are classified according to the *consciousnesses* who manifest in each one:

1. Troposphere *(Intraphysical): pre-serenissimus* or practitioners of penta who are *completely and permanently without intrusion;* assistential mini-pieces; assisted *intraphysical consciousnesses;* conscious and unconscious human *intruders.*

2. Para-troposphere *(Extraphysical):* assisted *extraphysical consciousnesses;* conscious and unconscious *extraphysical intruders;* unevolved *extraphysical communities;* assistential maxi-mechanism.

3. Evolved *extraphysical communities* (*Extraphysical*): *Helpers; evolutionary orientors;* assistential maxi-mechanism; *Serenissimus; Free Consciousnesses.*

22. ATTUNEMENT

Group. It is well known, in any human undertaking, that positive collective, group energy, or, even better, *consciential energy* coming from 1 cohesive, homogeneous group of *consciousnesses* transmitting with an effective sense of union and exceptional affinity, will manifest more intense and vigorous curative capacities that benefit the greatest number of receptive *consciousnesses*. This, as opposed to the isolated *consciential energy* derived from only 1 *consciousness*.

Audience. The artist in the limelight, the orator on the platform, the attorney in court, the professor behind the podium, and psychic individuals in altered states of *consciousness*, are familiar with the energy emanating from a *live audience*. From this was born the mediumistic or psychic session.

Attunement. The "psychic session of *I alone*" is apparently contrary to the principle referred to in the above mentioned group energy session. Nevertheless, the *penta practitioner is never alone*, as s/he acts in profound attunement with the *Helpers*, with healthy, self-aware *extraphysical consciousnesses* and, on rare occasions, even with projected *intraphysical consciousnesses* who are assisted by their *Helpers* and are functioning as *assistant-therapist to extraphysical consciousnesses*.

Supervision. The fact that *penta* is an animic-psychic task with only one person involved, facilitates the effectiveness and maintenance of supervision and energetic defense by the *Helpers*.

Maintenance. To begin an enterprise or destroy a work is easy. What is difficult, is the maintenance of an endeavor over time.

Union. When an attunement of *consciousnesses*, affinity of elevated sentiments, and cohesion in objectives is achieved, the relative percentage *of extraphysical* or *intraphysical consciousnesses* is not important. What counts is the union that creates the intensity of consciential energy that is mobilized with a cognizant, healthy, positive and *cosmoethical* intention.

Tasks. Included in the more elevated objectives of the *penta* practice is an increasing predomination of the assistential *clarification task*, as opposed to the assistential *consolation task*.

Success. Thus, we see that there are penta practices of greater or lesser quality, not only in terms of a particular practitioner in different periods of life, but, also, in the relative *interdimensional success* of different practitioners.

Singularity. He or she who experiences a singular or *peak* condition of greater responsibility in terms of self-knowledge, amidst the current terrestrial population, will inevitably, at the right or opportune time, embrace the practice of *penta*.

Conditions. The following 9 conditions can serve as units of measurement for the classification of the above-mentioned singularity:

1. Recognize your own *weak traits* and *strong traits*.
2. Look for a way out of your *consciential basement*.
3. Honor the *cosmoethic*.
4. Acknowledge the imperative of *maxi-fraternity* (mega-brotherhood).
5. Have taken an *intermissive course*.
6. Have a *macro-soma*.
7. Practice *existential inversion* or *existential recycling*.
8. Wish to amplify your *clarification task*.
9. Be aware of your *existential program*.

PENTA IS THE PERMANENT POST-GRADUATION COURSE OF THE CONSCIENTIOLOGIST.

Recycling. *Penta* is basic *assistential recycling* for the *intraphysical consciousness*.

Group of existential recyclers. Ideally, one day, the group of *existential recyclers* will be entirely composed of *penta practitioners*.

23. STAGES OF PENTA

Period. It is always intelligent to consider the existential period in which you live or the evolutionary level of the *penta practitioner.*

Stages. We can clearly see that there are 3 very distinct periods regarding the practices of *penta*:

1. Initial. The most difficult period or stage of *penta* – a practice that lasts for the rest of one's life – is the period of installation, which lasts for *6 months.*

2. Maintenance. The consolidation of the assistential-energetic practices of *penta* occurs within an average period of *3 years.*

3. Evolution. The evolved practice of *penta* – continuously, *at any time*, without mysticism and with one's *feet on the ground* and *mentalsoma* in the cosmos – generally occurs only after *1 decade* of daily exercises.

Specialization. In the evolved stage of *penta*, the practitioner can present specialized capacities. For example: the more frequent, healthy occurrence of a determinate psychic phenomenon; attending to *extraphysical consciousnesses* with specific lacks, with the support of a *Helper*, and others.

Micro-minority. Analyzing all the facts regarding this assistential practice, we can logically see why *penta* practitioners – nowadays in significant numbers – nonetheless still comprise an unquestionable micro-minority in the universe of lucid, human *projectors.*

24. ADVANCED STAGE OF PENTA

Synapses. *Penta* demands the creation of specific, high-quality neural synapses (neo-thosenes) due to the multidimensional or *holosomatic* nature of this process in the brain of the practitioner. This capacity is only obtained after a period of about 2 years.

Attributes. Upon greater analysis of the condition of one's own *consciousness*, the *penta practitioner* must see if s/he is going to be able to understand and utilize the following 6 of *his* or *her consciential* attributes:

1. Atemporality
2. Immateriality
3. Immortality
4. Inalienability
5. Objectivity
6. Rationality

Understanding. The evolution of *penta* demands that the practitioner understand the above-mentioned attributes.

Advanced. At an advanced stage, the practices of *penta* can be *extraphysically* oriented to have ectoplasmic effects. They will have the following 10 characteristics in their manifestations:

1. Dorsal. Employment of the dorsal position by the practitioner.
2. Temperature. Lowering of body and ambient temperature (ectoplasmy).
3. Effects. Agreeable psychic, *intraphysical* or bioenergetic phenomena (macro-PK).
4. *Soma*. Modification in the energetic exteriorizations pertaining to the *soma*, or rather: *more* energy transmitted from the trunk and head, and *less* from the arms and hands.

THE PRACTICE OF PENTA ALWAYS DEPENDS ON THE HEALTHY SOMA OF THE PRACTITIONER.

5. Respiration. Change in respiratory frequency during the energetic transmissions.
6. *Umbilical-chakra.* Obvious predominance in the activity of the *umbilical-chakra* in the energetic transmissions.
7. Abdomen. An upward pulling sensation through the abdomen with each energetic exteriorization.
8. Musculature. Strengthening of the abdominal muscles (the muscular mass becomes larger and more toned).
9. Metabolism. The practitioner's metabolism can undergo alterations, wherein s/he can feel an enhanced need for *glucose* (sugar), in certain cases; greater *diuresis*; or more *thirst,* resulting in an increased intake of liquids.
10. Hypertrophy. Cessation of the hypertrophy in the muscles of the arms and shoulders that was generated earlier through the intense movements used in the daily transmissions of energy.

Duration. Regarding the duration of the daily practice of *penta,* it is important to consider whether the energetic transmissions are *primary*, when located in the arms, or *evolved,* when focused in the thorax. In this sense, 2 variables become evident:

1. Arms. The transmissions of *consciential energies* in the practice of *penta* when the practitioner is seated, mostly employing the head, arms and hands, or rather: a predomination in the activity of the *coronal-chakra, frontal-chakra and laryngeal-chakra.* This is accomplished with faster, more pronounced, physical movements. The penta session, in this case, *is shorter.*
2. Thorax. The transmission of *consciential energies* in the practice of *penta,* wherein the practitioner is laying down and the thorax and abdomen are predominantly used, or rather: all 7 primary chakras are in action. This is done with slower, less intense physical movements. In this case, the penta session *is*

longer, and includes a greater frequency of ectoplasmic effects. All of this is relative, as everything depends on the psychological reactions of the practitioner in his or her *holosomatic* relationship with the *Helper*(s).

Semi-possession. As you can see, penta is a greater, continuous, omnipresent, healthy, conscious semi-possession on the part of the *Helper* during the assistential practice.

Camel. In this advanced stage of penta, the practitioner makes his or her reserves of ectoplasm available for greater energetic assistance at all times *(energetic para-metabolism)*, just as a camel uses its *hydric metabolism* in the desert.

Development. There are 2 types of development in the practice of penta, in terms of the specific, more predominant use of the basic chakras:

1. *Palm-chakras*. The practice of *elementary penta* is developed through the use of the practitioner's *2 palm-chakras*, behind which is located the *cardiochakra*. In this case, above all, the *classic holochakral circuit* occurs, being the most common with persons: *immanent energy* is absorbed through the sole-chakras and *consciential energy* is donated through the palm-chakras.

2. *Frontal-chakra*. In the *advanced* practice of *penta*, the *frontal-chakra* is used, above which is located the *coronal-chakra*.

Overvalue. the *penta practitioner, upon becoming a veteran*, no longer overvalues that which occurs with the great majority of the components of humanity, religions, conventional sciences, the arts, human ideologies in general and transitory intraphysical involvements in terms of one's own multidimensional realities that s/he has already identified, accepted, and now endeavors to experience.

Renovation. Your current life will never be the same as others' lives, or, more appropriately, will never be the same as your earlier lives or the lives of other human *consciousnesses*, in regards to the ideal, consensual and intelligent priority regarding evolution. This is a personal renovation and is, in fact, substantial, visceral and *surgical* in nature.

Yield. The intellectual and affective studies and speculations in the vast area of theory, philosophy, poetry and ideology, yield their place or *consciential* space, for the *penta practitioner* who experiences that which is priority for his or her evolution at the *present time*.

Para-synapses. The veteran *penta* practitioner's prioritized understanding of self and others is based in his or her permanent conquests, or, more specifically, those conquests within the *holo-memory*, in the *para-synapses* of the *para-brain*.

THE PARA-SYNAPSES ACT DIRECTLY IN THE HOLOSOMA OF THE PRACTITIONER BY WAY OF THE MENTALSOMA.

25. ADVANTAGES OF PENTA

Practicality. Daily *penta* exercises are extremely practical in regards to *intraphysical life*.

Advantages. Even an *intraphysical consciousness* who has individual, social commitments and is *not* even *able* to exercise his or her psychic capacities *twice* a week in a group of specialized practical studies, can practice penta and achieve the following 14 evident advantages, among others:

1. Regularity. *Penta* can be practiced every day.

2. Isolation. The practitioner's *penta* task can always be performed when s/he is alone, from a spatial *or intraphysical* point of view.

3. Discretion. The tasks can be maintained in secrecy, as there is neither the presence of a witness, nor the participation of other *intraphysical consciousnesses* or subhuman animals involved in the practitioner's *laboratory*.

4. Uninhibited. Excessive self-censure is eliminated, as the practitioner is isolated, with his or her thosenic processes, in his or her own experiences or manifestations.

5. Time. All of the work can occur outside of work time, work days or holidays, and planned social or professional, human obligations.

6. Locale. Everything occurs in the intimacy of one's own home or apartment; in a singular, welcome place – *one's own energetic field* – chosen by the practitioner-*Helper* duo on a permanent basis.

7. Residence. The performance of the penta task occurs without any driving or transit problems, which naturally avoids *psychic mishaps* in the hours prior to the daily practices.

8. Informality. The conventions, etiquette, ceremony and laws of a still pathological society – that often act as excessive components of the *steam roller of useless issues* – are completely eliminated.

9. Independence. This *interconsciential* assistance is executed independent of the critical judgment of the individuals in one's *evolutionary group*. This naturally avoids undesirable

egotistical *intrusions* between *intraphysical consciousnesses.*
The *penta practitioner* has to be self-sufficient in his or her life.
    10. Self-evident. The basic tenets of *Conscientiology*
recommend that everything that a *consciousness* affirms as theory be manifest in his or her life by his or her actions. It is only
reasonable to accept things based on the combined theory and
experience of universal phenomena reacting within a person.
Holomaturity begins with this essential measure. The experience
of *penta* permits a unique level of self-evidence.
    11. Proof. The practice of *penta* exercises offers the
practitioner the following 7 definitive proofs, among others:

    1. Existence of the *psychosoma.*
    2. Existence of the *holochakra.*
    3. Experience of the **multi-dimensionality** of *con-
sciousness.*
    4. Experience of the *lucid projectability* of *intra-
physical consciousness.*
    5. Consciousness' **survival** of *de-soma.*
    6. Experience of more evolved **psychic capacities.**
    7. Existence of and assistential coexistence with a
Helper.

    12. Gratification. *Penta* yields an indirect, multi-
dimensional evolutionary gratification.

PENTA IS AN ASSISTENTIAL UNDERTAKING WITH EXCEPTIONAL EVOLUTIONARY RESULTS.

    13. *Business venture.* Penta, when regarded as an *assis-
tential business venture,* is obviously the best type of evolutionary *franchising,* with the multi-dimensional team, for the individual. You give 1 hour of assistance every day to needy
extraphysical and *intraphysical consciousnesses,* and receive 23
hours of intraphysical and *extraphysical* energetic assistance

from the *Helpers* for the rest of your human existence. This can be shown in another manner with the following *formula:*

23 X 1 (or 100%) = 23 (or 2,300 %), or rather,

1/24 or 4.17% *effort* yields 23/24 or 95.83% *support*

PENTA IS A LANDMARK IN THE LIFE OF THE PRACTITIONER: BEFORE AND AFTER PENTA.

14. Landmark. *Penta* serves as a landmark in the existence of the practitioner, which becomes divided into 2 periods – *before penta* and *after penta* – due to the change for the better in one's personal *holothosene.* This includes 3 geographic and *para-geographic* realities that sustain the multi-dimensional practices:

1. *Physical base* – specifically geographical.
2. Energetically shielded space – geographical and *para-geographical.*
3. *Extraphysical clinic* – specifically *para-geographical.*

---
26. SUBTLETIES

Subtleties. Continuous *penta* presents a *paradox of subtle and ostentatious facets of* healthy *interconsciential assistentiality.* This is perceived through innumerous and very personal indications that are experienced, but are difficult to explain. It also, simultaneously presents the subtle and ostentatious facets of *pathological intrusion,* that is perceived through simple objects. For example: the narrow-minded individual being assisted who is wearing a blouse with a deep-sea-diving-suit print (in this case the shirt print was indicative that the consciousness was completely blocked or shielded to any incoming information); potted plants charged with pathological *consciential energy* that can be perceived at a distance.

Complexities. Evidently, these *simple* facts or silent messages, although having immense significant content only for the one who experiences them, are very *complex* in the analysis of their greater transcendence. Only *the* veteran *penta practitioner* can comprehend these extremely personal details.

Spontaneity. He or she who initiates penta should not concern themselves over these *subtle-complex* paradoxes. It is better to let them arise spontaneously over time and the accumulation of assistential experiences. Nevertheless, it would be intelligent to register the facts, dates, and circumstances involved, as well as the healthy consequences of everything that occurs in order to help the practitioner evolve in his or her awareness of the energetic-animic-psychic signals, or *impressive psychic capacities,* and the sophistication of the assistential monitoring that he or she will constantly receive.

Variables. In the *penta* practice, the following variables, among others, are of great interest: *auric coupling; physical base;* installed energetic field; brain; *cosmo-consciousness;* day-to-day *cosmoethical behavior,* being *completely and permanently without intrusion,* energetic dimension; *lucid energizer; consciential epicenter, holosomatic homeostasis; organic homeostasis; multidimensionality; extraphysical clinic; para-brain; psychic abilities in general; bioenergetic signals; holochakral looseness; terrestrial troposphere; lucid alternating life; energetic life.*

27. DAILY HABITS

Habits. The 5 following *daily* habits are recommended, with good reason, in the administration of the practice of *penta*, as well as being a manner in which to develop one's self-knowledge through *Conscientiology:*

1. Clothes. Change your *personal clothes* every day (sociability).
2. Bath. Take a *bath* every day (daily session of bodily *hygiene*).
3. Meals. Eat meals – and at least one *hot meal* – every day (survival of the soma).
4. Sex. Have *sex* every day (daily *sexual* session). This has to do with the existential implications of the most intimate, intraphysical *energetic contact* with another *intraphysical consciousness.*
5. *Penta.* Practice *penta* every day (daily *assistential* session). This has to do with the most intimate, multi-dimensional *energetic contact* with another *extraphysical consciousness* – the *Helper* – and other, assisted, *consciousnesses.*

Addiction. Regarding the practice of daily sex – which, according to statistics, is maintained by 10% of the population of the city of Sao Paulo, Brazil – the words of the Brazilian writer *Erico Verissimo* are worth recalling:

"The worst sexual addiction is abstinence."

28. NUDITY

Nudity. Given that the practice of penta is executed by a person exteriorizing *consciential energy* while alone, one can become psychically passive for the *Helpers* while physically naked with complete naturality, as long as one makes sure that there are no *drafts* in the room, the ambient *temperature* is adequate, and the *air conditioner* is properly used to avoid catching a cold. This allows one to overcome 2 factors:

1. *Helpers.* The *Helpers* have an evolved consciential nature, analyzing life through the lens of multi-dimensionality. They employ the *psychosoma*, and are not disturbed by the nudity of the practitioner.

2. Assisted. However, the practitioner's nudity can affect the reactions of the assisted *extraphysical consciousnesses* having either a masculine or feminine appearance, who are ill, tropospheric, *psychotic post-mortems*, or who *extraphysically* awaken due to the energy that is being transmitted in *penta*. These *consciousnesses* are still profoundly involved by *intraphysical* conditionings, repressions, *brain-washings*, narrow mindedness and sanctification.

29. *SYMPATHETIC ASSIMILATIONS*

Sympathetic assimilations. Sympathetic assimilations due to affinity, good intention, energetic predominance of illnesses, or disturbances of certain *intraphysical patients*, can occur in the energetic transmission of *penta.* This can be conscious or unconscious on the part of both the *assimilator-practitioner* and the *assimilated-patient.*

Remission. The definitive remission of symptoms in the *intraphysical* patient, after a period of hours, days, or even weeks of energetic transmissions, is what reveals, in many cases, the occurrence of *sympathetic assimilations.*

Cause. Whenever they occur, these *sympathetic assimilations* are benign, without negative consequences or bad intentions. They are provoked by the *Helpers* with the intention of promoting greater individual possibilities for the discarding of disturbances through the *energetic strengthening* of the energetic-psychic practitioner. The veteran transmitter can identify the *sympathetic assimilation* as soon as it is installed.

Immunization. Up to what point is the energetic strengthening or *protective aura* acquired by the *penta practitioner* a type of immunization? It serves as an immunization against poisons and is acquired through the absorption of small, gradually increasing, doses of the poison. Facts indicate that the veteran *penta practitioner* becomes *immunized,* with accumulated experiences over a decade, for example. In other words, he or she becomes immunized against the ill, *consciential energy* of *intruders.* This furthers the practitioner's progress towards the condition of being *completely and permanently without intrusion.* Energetic immunization that is acquired in assistential service is the decisive first step needed for an *intraphysical consciousness* to become liberated from the serial nature of human existences *(rebirth cycle).*

THE PRACTICE OF PENTA DOES NOT PRODUCE ENERGETIC HANGOVERS.

Disturbances. Following is a typical example of *sympathetic assimilation* with the pathological conditions of the *somaholochakra-psychosoma* of an ill *intraphysical consciousness*: someone has problems in his or her leg, for example, that has been exhibiting pain, swelling, difficulty in walking, and other disturbances. The individual has already undergone all possible examinations, diagnoses and useless conventional therapies. The disturbances then disappear with the energetic transmissions of penta, including those performed at a distance.

Bait. *Sympathetic assimilation* is the most advanced assistential condition of animic-psychic consciential bait. It is based on 3 factors:

1. State of *rapport* or affinity.
2. Existence of *consciential energies*.
3. Phenomenon of *auric coupling*.

Therapeutic. The *intrusion*, in this case, is not an episode of *interconsciential intrusion* as we understand it. The occurrence is, above all, therapeutic and not pathological. It does, however, in a great number of cases, arise from chronic *intrusion* and the syncretic practices of many sects.

Responsory. The practices popularly called *responses* and *responsories* are positively executed through the *sympathetic assimilation* of *consciential energy*.

Fire. The *penta practitioner* need not fear being locked in his or her room during a catastrophe − a fire in the building, for example. The *Helpers* are alert to any irregularity inside or outside of the location of penta and will advise the practitioner in time. The experience of *penta* evidences this fact.

30. *EVOLUTION OF CONSCIOUSNESS*

Scale. Following is an evolutionary scale of the *assistential consciousness* of human personality, according to *Conscientiometry* (measurement of *consciousness*):

1. *Pre-serenissimus.* Vulgar, *pre-serenissimus intra-physical consciousness* having a mediocre existential program and no fixed residence.
2. *Mini-intrusion.* Common, eventual *mini-intrusions*, in terms of *interconsciential assistentiality.*
3. Practitioner. *Self-organized penta practitioner.*
4. Bait. Aware *assistential bait.*
5. Sensitive. High quality psychic sensitive.
6. *Extraphysical clinic.* Has a fixed residence and is responsible for an extraphysical clinic.
7. *Consciential epicenter.* Aware *consciential epicenter* with a perceptible energetic field permanently installed as a small cog of a large assistential mechanism.
8. *Completely and permanently without intrusion.*
9. *Completist.* One who has executed a greater *existential program (existential mega-program).*
10. *Existential moratorium* recipient. Conscious recipient of a greater *existential moratorium (existential maxi-moratorium).*

Will. *Penta* is neither a cure-all nor a universal panacea. For example, penta does not vaccinate the practitioner against corruption. *The penta practitioner's* will and intention vaccinate him or her against corruption.

31. CONSCIENTIAL BALANCE

Synthesis. Synthesizing this text up to this point, we arrive at some thoughts and conclusions.

Evolution. To evolve is to completely domesticate and employ immanent energy with greater intelligence.

THE PRACTITIONER IS FIRST AND MOST GREATLY BENEFITED BY THE PRACTICE OF PENTA.

Para-professional. The *penta practitioner* is a *para-professional* of *interconsciential assistentiality*. If we wish to establish a comparison between individuals – in view of the seriousness and depth of the *intraphysical* and *extraphysical* engagement demanded by the processes of *penta* – we can say that all assistential *human consciousnesses* who do not practice *penta* are merely *amateurs.*

Mega-loyalty. One of the salient points in the development of *penta* is the permanent *maximal loyalty, above everything and all other loyalties,* or the perseverant and abnegate dedication as an *intra*physical *mini*-piece to the *extra*physical assistential *maxi*-mechanism. This, without becoming alienated from the obligations of daily human life, and without fanaticism, veneration, guru-worship or elitism. Regarding the small-cog-large-mechanism dynamic, it is good to remember: *a whale, as big as it is, remains microscopic in the vastness of the ocean.*

Obligations. Being a path with no return, penta is a stronger and more rigorous obligation than *traditional marriage,* or the *evolutionary duo.* Penta does not allow divorce. For example: it is easier to be a champion at boxing – a radical, violent and condemnable sport – than to practice high-quality *penta.*

Conscientiotherapy. Penta dots the "i"s, goes to the bone, and anatomizes the *consciousness* of the practitioner. *Penta* is an *encyclopedia of self-knowledge* as well as being *self-* and *hetero-conscientiotherapy.*

Images. *Penta* goes beyond the most transcendent images, dreams and perspectives that are yearned for by the *human consciousness.*

Behavior. *Penta* is the most challenging, evolved, paradoxical or apparently ambiguous of all the types of behavior that the aware *intraphysical consciousness* can propose or dedicate itself to.

PENTA IS THE MOST EGOCENTRIC-ALTRUISTIC INTRAPHYSICAL PARADOXICAL PRACTICE THAT EXISTS.

Light. There is no *light* version of *penta* – nor would it work. All of its practices are clearly defined, without obscurity, misinterpretations or possible side-tracks. *Anti-cosmoethical* behavior in the practice of *penta* is a mechanism of inexorable evolutionary self-destruction.

Island. The *penta practitioner* represents an island of organized efficiency in the sea of *interconsciential* and multidimensional assistentiality.

Total. It is calculated – as a supposition – that there are, now in 1995, *hundreds of active penta practitioners.* This is a hypothetical number. It is difficult to affirm anything of this nature with relative assurance so far, in view of our restricted statistical micro-universe.

Solitude. The practice of *penta* ends any type of solitude on the part of the practitioner. He or she will always be in the *good company* of the *Helpers.*

---
32. THEORY OF THE ABUNDANCE OF
CONSCIENTIAL ENERGY

Question. A pertinent question fits well here: Why is the practice of *penta* possible today, but was not common or more easily executed in humanity's past? *Conscientiology* has a rational response for this question, based on *intraphysical* and multi-dimensional facts.

Abundance. We live today, on Earth, in a unique situation, that has still not been detected outside of *Conscientiology*, or evidenced in life. This condition supports the *theory of the abundance of consciential energy*, proposed by this author.

Mini-connections. The *abundance* of *consciential energy* is explained by the increase, as never before, in the number of mini-connections of energetic flows (see ch. 11), or the connections of *holochakras* with somas, through the population explosion that, by the end of 1994, showed a planetary population of 5.650 billion human beings, or more conscious individuals, spread over the crust of this planet (representing 5.650 billion mini-connections of *holochakras* with *somas*).

Viability. This *abundance or potentiation of consciential energy* created a vigorous energetic *holothosene* that predisposes the possibility of *interconsciential* assistance and makes the broadening of the practice of *penta* viable.

Population. The population explosion also opened channels for the spreading and greater use of *penta.*

Matter. As well, the increase in the number of mini-connections of *holochakras* in somas has amplified the existing volume of *matter that has been energized* by consciousnesses in intraphysical life on Earth.

Holothosene. The increased volume and higher quality of energized matter has improved the *planetary holothosene* of Earth and *intraphysical life*, as well as further predisposing the appearance of *cosmoethical*, more advanced psychic phenomena, including the following 10:

1. A great diversity of intellectually gifted individuals (prodigies and precocious children).

2. Psychically gifted individuals (bioenergetic, animic and psychic capacities).

3. Incidence of healthy, high quality ectoplasmic phenomena, without spectacular exhibitions.

4. Therapeutic and *extraphysical clinical* phenomena.

5. Psychic surgery.

6. *Para-anesthesia.*

7. *Para-asepsis.*

8. *Para-hemostasis.*

9. *Para-scarring.*

10. Appearance and disappearance of large and small objects in space-time-matter.

Theory. Even from the succinct examples given here, one can logically conclude that the theory of abundance of consciential energy is capable of fulfilling the 7 basic requirements demanded by the rigors of science as qualities necessary for a theory, or rather:

1. Methodology: systematizes human understanding in regards to the energies of *consciousness.*

2. Concepts: serves as a source for the analytical structuring of concepts and conceptual classification (system of reference).

3. Facts: explains, generalizes and synthesizes the understanding of problems and phenomena (facts).

4. Knowledge: increases mankind's knowledge and discovers gaps indicating areas that have still not been explored in this area of mankind's understanding (bioenergetics).

5. Contrastability: strengthens the contrastability or contributes towards the verification of factual, veridical values.

6. Research: orients conscientiological research.

7. Route: offers a route for a sector of consciential reality and becomes a means for making previsions of facts.

33. EFFECTS OF PENTA

Effects. An obvious question is worth asking at this point in the considerations: what are the healthy effects from the practice of penta after 1 decade?

Evaluation. It is easy to evaluate the result of this effort, using the simple arithmetical example that follows:

50	min.	in	300	days (1 year with 65 days subtracted)
15,000	min.	in	1	year (300 days)
150,000	min.	in	10	years (1 decade or 3,000 days)
2,500	hours	in	1	decade
104	days	in	1	decade
3.5	months	in	1	decade
1/40	life	in	4	decades

Subtraction. The subtracting of 65 days (obviously exaggerated in order to achieve round numbers) represents practically inevitable illnesses and natural impediments to the practice of penta exercises during the 12 months of the year. Examples of natural impediments: an illness of someone close to you; a domestic problem; an unexpected trip that cannot be postponed; unexpected professional demands; facts that cannot be rationally attributed to or interpreted as psychic mishaps.

Beach. We can compare penta with other activities. A leisure activity such as going to the beach, for example, demands much more of our time than penta and offers almost no *great* benefit in regards to our evolution – aside from skin cancer generated from sunning oneself between 10:00 a.m. and 3:00 p.m.

Decades. The 3.5 months of continuous assistential energetic practice, or a 3.5 month immersion of *extraphysical* prime time over 1 decade, as calculated above, can take place, for example, from 30 to 40 years of age, from 40 to 50, or from 50 to 60 years of physical age. If one practices *penta* from 30 to 70 years of physical age – 4 decades – they will donate *1 entire year* of their life to assistentiality, or 1/40 of this 4 decades of *intraphysical life*. This does not take into account other inevitable multi-dimensional participation: conscious projections during nightly periods of natural sleep, for example.

Extra time. We also did not add in the extra time that is required in preparation, *holosomatic warm-up*, and *mental and somatic connections* to *extra*physical life. Also, *after* the daily exercise, the time required for *re*-entry into intraphysical life was not considered.

Veteran. However there is more than this, as the *veteran practitioner* responds to the need for exteriorizations of assistential energy at any time of the day or night.

Leader. It is impractical to calculate the number of *consciousnesses* attended during daily *penta* exercises. It is enough to consider the hypothesis of treating only 1 *pathological extraphysical leader* who influences 1,200 imbalanced *consciousnesses* – which sometimes occurs in pathological *extraphysical communities*. How can we know the results of this assistance? Perhaps only after our de-soma, together with the *Evolutionary Orientor*.

34. POTENT FORCES

Forces. Following are the 8 *most potent* forces of *those-nic* manifestation by *consciousness* in *intraphysical life*, in order of decreasing intensity:

1. Will. Iron-clad *will* (volition).
2. Intentionality. The control of *maxi-fraternal, cosmo-ethical intentionality* (intention).
3. Self-organization. *Multi-dimensional self-organization* relative to *intraphysicality, bioenergetics, mentalsomatics* and psychic capacities *(consciential* self-mastery).
4. Penta. *Penta* practiced through assistential bioenergetics at a high level of maturity.
5. *Extraphysical clinic.* A fully functioning *extraphysical clinic*, predisposing the consciential epicenter to an *existential moratorium*, if appropriate.
6. *Evolutionary duo.* Active participation in an intimate *evolutionary duo.*
7. Mega-gestations. *Consciential mega-gestations* (developments) executed individually, in an *evolutionary duo*, or in group.
8. *Existential project.* An *existential project* in steady development, proceeding towards *existential completism.*

Powers. These 8 forces are the truest and most relevant powers that an *intraphysical consciousness* can avail him or herself to.

Values. These 8 forces are the *most important* values needed in order for an aware *intraphysical consciousness* to accelerate his or her lucid evolution.

Placement. It is important to reflect with maximum hetero-criticism over the vitally logical placement of penta in *fourth place* on this list.

Discernment. Discernment or good common sense gained by the practitioner's experience is the best indicator for the improvement or incessant development in the practice of *penta.*

STRICTLY SPEAKING, ONLY LACK OF COURAGE IS INCURABLE.

Weakness. Weakness (in this case, lack of motivation, neediness, abulia or lack of will) is the path towards all pathologies and *para-pathologies* of *consciousness.*

Personal. I am, personally, completely available to each and every individual interested in practicing *penta*, within my limited *intraphysical* possibilities and in the confessed condition of being a *merchant of my own literate ignorance* regarding the themes of *consciousness*, which are of a higher priority than all others at our current evolutionary stage.

GLOSSARY OF CONSCIENTIOLOGY

Observations. Following are listed 282 denominations, neologisms, expressions and their technical equivalents in *Conscientiology.*

Advanced existential program – *Existential program* of an *intraphysical consciousness* who is an evolutionary leader, performing within a specific libertarian *group-karmic* task that is more universalist and poly-karmic in nature. This individual serves as a lucid, *mini-*cog acting within a *maxi-*mechanism of a multi-dimensional team.

Alternate intraphysical pre-serenissimus – *Intraphysical consciousness* capable of simultaneously living consciously in the waking state as well as projected in the extraphysical dimensions, from time-to-time.

Andro-chakra (*andro* + *chakra*) – A man's *sex-chakra.*

Andro-thosene (neologism: *andro* + *tho* + *sen* + *ene*) – *Thosene* of the primitive masculine or *macho* man.

Animism (Latin: *animus,* soul) – Set of *intra-* and *extracorporeal* phenomena produced by the *intraphysical consciousness* without external interference. Example: the phenomenon of *conscious projection* induced by one's own will.

Anti-thosene (*anti* + *tho* + *sen* + *ene*) – Antagonistic *thosene,* common in refutations, omni-questionings and in productive debates.

Aphrodisiac feminine sex-soma – *Soma* of a woman, specifically when considered in regards to sex, when having an appearance that is capable of acting as an aphrodisiac. See *gynosoma.*

Assisted conscious projection – Projection wherein a *consciousness* finds him or herself directly assisted during the experience by a *Helper* who is almost always an expert in lucid *projectability.*

Auric coupling – Interfusion of *holochakral* energies between 2 or more *consciousnesses.*

Belly-brain – *Abdominal sub-brain,* the *umbilical-chakra* (center of *consciential energy* located above the navel), when unconsciously selected by an *intraphysical consciousness*, who is still at a mediocre stage of evolution, for the task of basing his or her manifestations upon. The *belly-brain, abdominal brain, abdominal pseudo-brain*, or *abdominal sub-brain*, is a *parody* of the natural, encephalic brain (*coronal-chakra* and *frontal-chakra*); an indefensible embarrassment in conscious self-evolution.

Biothosene (*bio + tho + sen + ene*) – *Thosene* specifically related to *human consciousness*.

Brady-thosene (*brady + tho + sen + ene*) – *Thosene* having a sluggish flow, pertaining to the slow-minded *human consciousness*.

Cardio-chakra (*cardio + chakra*) – The fourth basic chakra; influential agent in the emotionality of an *intraphysical consciousness*; vitalizes the heart and lungs; heart chakra.

Chakra – A nucleus or defined field of *consciential energy*. The totality of the many chakras in one's energetic system constitutes the *holochakra* or *energetic para-body*. The *holochakra*, inside the *soma*, forms a junction between the *soma* and *psychosoma*, acting as a point of connection through which *consciential energy* flows from one *vehicle* to another.

Chirosoma (*chiro + soma*) – The body considered specifically in regards to the use of hands or manual work.

Clarification task – Advanced personal or group task of enlightenment or clarification.

Con – Hypothetical unit of measure of the lucidity of an *intraphysical* or *extraphysical consciousness*.

Conscientese – Telepathic non-symbolic idiom that is native to the *consciential dimensions* of very evolved *extraphysical* societies.

Consciential amentia – Condition in which a *consciousness* is incapable of thinking with reasonable mental balance.

Consciential basement – Phase of infantile and adolescent manifestations of *intraphysical consciousness* up until adulthood, characterized by a predominance of the more primitive weak traits of *consciousness* – *consciousness* being multi-vehicular, multi-existential and multi-millenary.

Consciential concentration – The direct, unswerving, focusing of one's senses, *consciential* attributes, will and intention upon a singular object.

Consciential continuism – Condition of continuity of *consciential* life through preview and evolutionary self-alternation, or rather: the incessant correction of one's experience of the present moment, those immediately anterior and posterior, in a cohesive and unified whole, without loss of continuity or impervious *consciential* experiences; condition of being lucid from lifetime to lifetime, including when your body is asleep, etc.

Consciential dermatological (superficial) approaches – Compound expression attributed to the conventional, physicalist sciences that are subordinated to the newtonian-cartesian, mechanistic paradigm, and focus their research only on the soma – not availing themselves to the instrumentation necessary for the direct, technical investigation of *consciousness* itself; dermatological approaches of *intraphysical consciousness*. *Periconsciential* sciences.

Consciential ectopia – Unsatisfactory execution of one's *existential program* in an eccentric, dislocated manner, outside the programming chosen for the individual's *intraphysical life*.

Consciential energy – *Immanent energy* that a *consciousness* employs in its general manifestations; the *ene* of *thosene*; personal energy.

Consciential epicenter – Key *intraphysical consciousness* who becomes a fulcrum of interdimensional lucidity, assistentiality and constructiveness through the use of the *extraphysical clinic*. Directly related to *penta* or personal energetic task.

Consciential era – That era in which the average *intraphysical consciousness* finds him or herself sufficiently evolved, through impacts, personal redefinition and revolutions created through experiences of *lucid projectability*, to implant the *priority of self-conscientiality*.

Consciential eunuch – Individual *conscientially* castrated and manipulated by the sectarian domesticators of *satisfied human automatons (robots)*, who are modern slaves of the unthinking masses.

Consciential gestation – Evolutionary productivity on the part of an *intraphysical consciousness* in terms of the execution of its *existential program*.

Consciential hyperspace – *Extraphysical consciential* dimensions.

Consciential micro-universe – *Consciousness* when considered as a whole, including all of its attributes, *thosenes* and manifestations in its evolution. The microcosmos of *consciousness* in relation to the macrocosmos of the universe.

Consciential mono-capability – *Intraphysical life* under the pressure of constant *intrusions* by ill beings. This is experienced by mediocre *intraphysical consciousnesses* having few talents and no versatility.

Consciential para-comatose – State of *extraphysical* coma of a *projected intraphysical consciousness*, who invariably remains unconscious and, therefore, has no recall of *extraphysical* events.

Consciential paradigm – Leading-theory of *Conscientiology*, founded in *consciousness* itself.

Consciential retailing – A rudimentary system of individual behavior characterized by lesser, isolated *consciential* actions having a minimum of productive results or important evolutionary effects.

Consciential scaffolds – Dispensable psychological or physical *crutches* used by *consciousness*.

Consciential self-bilocation (Latin: *bis*, two; and *locus*, place) – Act whereby an *intraphysical projector* encounters and contemplates his or her own human body (*soma*) face-to-face, when his or her *consciousness* is outside of the *soma* (in the case of an *intraphysical consciousness*) and in another vehicle of *consciential* manifestation.

Consciential tri-capability – Quality of the 3 talents most useful to *conscientiology* – intellectuality, psychic abilities and communicability – when found together.

Consciential wholesaling – Behavior of an individual characterized by a tendency to approach issues in a comprehensive or wholesale manner so as not to leave negative evolutionary loose ends or *gaps* behind.

Conscientiocentric institution – That institution which centralizes its objectives on *consciousness* and its evolution, as is the case with the International Institute of Projectiology and Conscientiology (IIPC); *consciential* cooperative, within *Consci-*

entiological Society, having employment and *consciential* ties at its foundation.

　Conscientiogram – Technical plan for evaluative measurement of the evolutionary level of *consciousness; consciential mega-test* having *Homo sapiens serenissimus* as a model – *Serenissimus* being responsible for a positive *ego-karmic account.* The *conscientiogram* is the basic instrument employed in *conscientiometric* tests.

　Conscientiologist – *Intraphysical consciousness* engaged in the continuing study and objective experimentation in the field of *conscientiology* research. The *conscientiologist* operates as an agent of evolutionary renovation (*retrocognitive agent*), in the liberating work of *consciousnesses* in general.

　Conscientiology – Science that studies *consciousness* in an integral, *holosomatic,* multi-dimensional multi-millenary, multi-existential manner and, overall, according to its reactions with regards to immanent energy, *consciential energy* and its own multiple states of being.

　Conscientiometry – Discipline that studies *consciential* measurements through the use of resources and methods offered by *Conscientiology,* capable of establishing the possible bases of the *mathematical analysis of consciousness.* The *conscientiogram* is the principle instrument used in *conscientiometry.*

　Conscientiotherapy – Treatment, alleviation or remission of disturbances of *consciousness* executed through the resources and techniques derived from *Conscientiology.*

　Conscious projection (CP) – Projection of *an intraphysical consciousness* beyond the soma; extracorporeal experience; out-of-body experience (OBE).

　Consolation task – A primary-level personal or group *assistential task of consolation.*

　Coronal-chakra (*coronal + chakra*) – Chakra at the top of the head, crowning the *holochakra;* crown chakra.

　Cosmo-consciousness – Condition of a *consciousness'* inner awareness of the cosmos, of life and the order of the universe, in an intellectual and *cosmoethical* exaltation that is impossible to describe. In this case, a *consciousness* senses the living presence of the universe around him or her, in an indivisible unity. *Interconsciential* communication occurs in this peculiar condition.

Cosmoethic (*cosmo + ethic*) – Ethic or reflection over the cosmic, multi-dimensional morality that defines *holomaturity*. Cosmoethic is situated beyond the social, intraphysical morality, or that which presents itself to be beyond any human label.

Cosmoethical mimicry – Productive social impulse towards imitation of one's evolved forebears.

Cosmoethicality – A *consciousness' cosmoethic* nature.

Cosmothosene (*cosmo + tho + sen + ene*) – *Thosene* specifically related to *conscientese* or the state of *cosmoconsciousness*; form of communication of *conscientese*.

Co-thosene (*co + tho + sen + ene*) – *Thosene* specifically related to the collective actions of a chorus, of those praying in groups or crowds.

Counter-body – Same as *holochakra*, the vehicle of an *intraphysical consciousness' consciential energy;* energetic body.

Counter-thosene (*counter + tho + sen + ene*) – *Intraconsciential thosene* of an *intraphysical consciousness*; mute mental refutation; mental word; mute thosene; a type of *intra-thosene*.

Daydream – Fanciful story created by one's imagination during the waking state of *human consciousness*.

De-soma (*de + soma*) – *Somatic* deactivation, impending and inevitable for all *intraphysical consciousnesses*; final projection; *first death*; biological death; monothanatosis. De-soma (by itself) or *first de-soma* is the deactivation of the human body or *soma* (biological death). S*econd de-soma* is the deactivation of the *holochakra*. T*hird de-soma* is the deactivation of the *psychosoma*.

Destructive macro-PK – Harmful PK (*psychokinesis*) capable of causing losses to the *intraphysical consciousness*. Destructive macro-PK can prove fatal.

Domiciliary holo-thosene – Physical base; bedroom that has been energetically shielded; *extraphysical clinic*.

Dream – Natural *consciential* state that is intermediary between the waking state and natural sleep. Dreams are characterized by a set of ideas and images that present themselves to *consciousness*. An afflictive dream includes agitation, anguish and oppression in its development, and is known as: *nightmare; night terror; nightmarish hallucination.*

Ego-karma (*ego + karma*) – Principle of cause and effect acting in the evolution of *consciousness*, when centered exclusively around the ego per se. State wherein one's free will is restricted by infantile egocentrism.

Egothosene (*ego + tho + sen + ene*) – Same as *self-thosene*; *unit of measurement* of *consciential* egotism according to *Conscientiology* or, more appropriately, according to *Conscientiometry.*

Energetic dimension – Energetic dimension of *consciousnesses*; *holochakral* dimension; *third-and-a-half* dimension. Dimension natural to the *holochakra.*

Energetic intrusion – Invasion of an *intraphysical consciousness* by another using *consciential energies* or *holochakra*; *holo-chakral intrusion.*

Energetic maxi-spring – Condition of a maximized or prolonged *energetic spring* (energetic plenitude).

Energetic mini-spring – Condition of a minimal or ephemeral *energetic spring* (energetic plenitude).

Energetic spring – A more-or-less long-lasting condition wherein one's *consciential energies* exhibit an optimal, healthy, constructive profile.

Energetic spring by two – *Energetic spring* of an *evolutionary duo*, the partners of which truly love each other and have mastered the application of healthy consciential energy with complete lucidity, building their *existential program* through *consciential gestations.*

Enumerology – Didactic technique of processing texts based on informative self-critiquing.

Evolutionary duo – Two *consciousnesses* that interact positively in joint evolution; existential condition of *cooperative evolutionality* by two individuals.

Evolutionary orientor – *Consciousness* who is assistential in the intelligent coordination of an individual's *existential program*, or in the *consciential* evolution of one or more individuals in the same karmic group; *Helper;* Evolutionary condition in-between *Serenissimus* and the status of being *completely and permanently without intrusion.*

Existential completism – Condition of a *human consciousness' existential program* having been completed.

Existential inversion – Technique of optimizing one's *consciential* performance in the *preparatory phase* of the individual's *existential program* (up through 35 years of physical age).

Existential invertability – Quality of *intraphysical execution* of *existential inversion*.

Existential invertor – One who disposes him or herself to the execution of *existential inversion* in *intraphysical life*.

Existential maxi-moratorium – Condition of a greater *existential moratorium* or that which occurs for a *completist*, coming as an addition to his or her finished *existential program*; execution of a *healthy extension* to an *existential mandate* that has been concluded.

Existential maxi-program – *Maximal existential program* having a wholesale approach. It targets the execution of tasks of universalism and *maxi-fraternity* having *poly-karmic* bases.

Existential mini-moratorium – Condition of a lesser *existential moratorium* or that which occurs for an , coming as an opportunity to compensate for his or her holo-karmic *deficit* or to achieve the status of *completist regarding* his or her *existential program*; the finishing of a still incomplete *existential mandate*.

Existential mini-program – *Existential program* targeting the execution of a minimal, *group-karmic task*.

Existential moratorium – An extension of *intraphysical life* given to selected *intraphysical consciousnesses* according to their *holo-karmic merit*. An *existential moratorium* can be based on deficiency in (*existential mini-moratorium*) or completion of (*existential maxi-moratorium*) the individual's *existential program*.

Existential program – Specific program of each *intraphysical consciousness,* to be executed in their current *intraphysical life*.

Existential recyclability – Quality of the *intraphysical* execution of *existential recycling*.

Existential recycler – *Intraphysical consciousness* who disposes him or herself to the execution of *existential recycling*.

Existential recycling – Technique for the realization of one's *existential program*, executed by a *human consciousness*.

Existential robotization – Condition of a tropospheric *intraphysical consciousness* who is enslaved to *intraphysicality* or quadridimensionality.

Existential self-mimicry – Imitation of one's own past experiences, be they related to their *intraphysical* life or to previous *intraphysical* lives.

Existential seriation – 1. Evolutionary *existential seriation* of *consciousness*; successive existences; *intraphysical* rebirths in series. 2. *Intraphysical* or human life. Outworn synonym: *reincarnation*; this archaic word no longer serves those more serious individuals dedicated to leading-edge *consciousness* research.

Extraphysical – Relative to that which is outside, or beyond, the *intraphysical* or human state; *consciential* state *less physical* than the human body; non-physical.

Extraphysical agenda – written notes of priority *consciential extraphysical* targets – beings, locales or ideas – that the projected individual seeks to gradually reach, in a chronological manner, establishing intelligent plans for his or her development.

Extraphysical approach – Contact of a *consciousness* with another in the *extraphysical* dimensions.

Extraphysical catatonia – Fixed condition whereby a projected *intraphysical consciousness* performs stereotypical repetitive acts that are generally useless or dispensable in terms of his or her evolution.

Extraphysical clinic – *Extraphysical* treatment center of an *intraphysical epicenter* (*penta* practitioner); *extraphysical clinic*. The resources and *extraphysical installations* of the *extraphysical clinic* are numerous and remarkable. The *extraphysical clinic* is a domiciliary *holothosene.*

Extraphysical community – A common lifestyle setting of *extraphysical consciousnesses* in an *extraphysical* dimension.

Extraphysical Consciousness – *Para-citizen* of *extraphysical society*; disembodied *consciousness.* Outworn synonym: *discarnate.*

Extraphysical euphoria – Euphoria experienced after biological death due to the reasonably satisfactory completion of one's *existential program; post-mortem* euphoria; *para-euphoria*; *post-somatic euphoria.*

Extraphysical melancholy – Condition of *extraphysical, post-somatic or post-mortem melancholy; para-melancholy.*

Extraphysical monitoring – Condition wherein assistance is given by healthy *extraphysical consciousnesses* to a balanced *intraphysical consciousness,* when said individual is performing balanced tasks of consolation or clarification.

Extraphysical precognition (Latin: *pre,* before; *cognoscere,* know) – Perceptive faculty whereby a *consciousness,* while fully projected outside the human body, comes to know about indeterminate upcoming facts, as well as objects, scenes and distant forms, in the future.

Extraphysical romance – Totality of acts whereby an *intraphysical consciousness* maintains a healthy or positive romantic relationship while projected outside the body.

Extraphysical society – Society of *extraphysical consciousnesses.*

Free consciousness (Latin: *con + scientia,* with knowing) – *Extraphysical consciousness* who has definitively liberated him or herself *(deactivation)* from the *psychosoma* or emotional body and the web of existential seriation *(rebirth cycle). Free consciousness* is situated in the *evolutionary hierarchy* above *Homo sapiens serenissimus.*

Geo-energy (*geo + energy*) – *Immanent energy* deriving from the soil or earth and absorbed by an *intraphysical consciousness* through the *pre-kundalini* (sole) chakras. Archaic expression: *telluric energy.*

Golden cord – Supposed energetic element – similar to a remote control – that maintains the *mentalsoma* connected to the *extraphysical* brain of the *psychosoma.*

Grapho-thosene (*grapho + tho + sen + ene*) – The *thosenic signature* of a *human consciousness.*

Group of existential inverters – *Intraphysical consciousnesses* meeting together in groups, objectifying experimentation in planned *existential inversion.*

Group of existential recyclers – *Intraphysical consciousnesses* meeting together in groups, objectifying experimentation in planned existential recycling.

Groupality – Quality of the *evolutionary group* of a *consciousness;* condition of *group evolutionality.*

Group-karma (*group* + *karma*) – Principle of cause and effect acting in the evolution of *consciousness*, when pertaining to the *evolutionary group*. State wherein one's free will is bound to one's *evolutionary group*.

Group-karmic course – Sum total of stages (intraphysical lives) of *consciousness* wherein one is more closely tied to one's *consciential evolutionary group*.

Group-karmic inter-prison – Condition of *group-karmic* inseparability from an evolutionary *consciential* principle or from a specific *consciousness*.

Group-thosene – A sectarian, corporate, *anti-poly-karmic thosene*. A *group-thosene* can also be constructive.

Gyno-chakra (*gyno* + *chakra*) – *Sex-chakra* of a woman.

Gyno-soma (*gyno* + *soma*) – The female human body, specialized in the animal reproduction of *intraphysical consciousness* in *intraphysical life;* aphrodisiac body.

Gyno-thosene (*gyno* + *tho* + *sen* + *ene*) – *Thosene* specifically related to feminine language and communicability.

Hallucination (Latin: *hallucinari*, to err) – Apparent perception of an external object that is not present in the moment; mental error in one's sensory perceptions which are not founded in objective reality.

Helper – *Extraphysical consciousness* that assists or serves as an auxiliary to one or more *intraphysical* consciousnesses; *extraphysical* benefactor. Outworn equivalent expressions: *guardian angel; angel of light; angel; mentor; spirit guide*.

Hetero-thosene (*hetero* + *tho* + *sen* + *ene*) – The *thosene* of another in relation to ourself.

Holo-chakra (*holo* + *chakra*) – *Extraphysical energetic body* of *human consciousness*. Sum total of all chakras in one's energetic system; energetic double; energetic body; pranic body.

Holochakral existence – *Intraphysical life* or the existential seriation of the *intraphysical existences* of *human consciousness*.

Holochakral intrusion – Invasion of an *intraphysical consciousness* by another using the *holo-chakra* or *consciential energies; energetic intrusion*.

Holochakral looseness – Condition of relative freedom of action of the *energetic para-body* of an *intraphysical consciousness*, as compared to its *psychosoma* and *soma.*

Holochakral seduction – Energetic action of one *consciousness* over another (or others) with a more-or-less conscious intention of domination.

Holo-chakrality – Qualities of the manifestations of *intraphysical consciousness* deriving from the *holochakra.*

Holo-karma (*holo* + *karma*) – The 3 types of *consciential* actions and reactions – *ego-karma, group-karma* and *poly-karma* – within the acting principles of cause and effect in evolution of *consciousness. Ego-karma, group-karma* and *poly-karma* when considered as a whole.

Holomaturity (*holo* + *maturity*) – Condition of the integrated maturity – biological, psychological, *holosomatic* and multi-dimensional – of *human consciousness.*

Holomemory (*holo* + *memory*) – Causal, compound, multi-millenary, multi-existential, implacable, uninterrupted, personal memory that retains all facts relative to *consciousness;* multi-memory; poly-memory.

Holo-orgasm (*holo* + *orgasm*) – *Holosomatic* orgasm; maximum ecstasy generated through the energy of the entire *holosoma.*

Holosoma *(holo* + *soma*) – Set of vehicles of manifestation of *intraphysical consciousness: soma, holochakra, psychosoma* and *mentalsoma;* set of vehicles of manifestation of *extraphysical consciousness: psychosoma* and *mentalsoma.*

Holosomatic homeostasis – Integrated, healthy state of harmony of the *holosoma.*

Holosomatic interfusion – State of maximal *sympathetic assimilation* between 2 *consciousnesses.*

Holosomatic intrusion – Invasion of an *intraphysical consciousness* by another using the entire *holosoma.*

Holosomatics – Discipline that studies the *holosoma.*

Holo-thosene (*holo* + *tho* + *sen* + *ene*) – Aggregated or consolidated *thosenes.* This word generates resistance in a wide band of serious readers of the sciences.

Homo sapiens serenissimus – A *consciousness* that is integrally experiencing its condition of lucid serenism; a *con-*

sciousness that is about to pass through the third de-soma (end of rebirth cycle). Popular synonym: *Serenissimus.*

Homo-thosene *(homo + tho + sen + ene)* – The *thosene* of telepathic emission and reception; the *unit of measurement* in telepathy according to *Conscientiology.*

Hyper-acuity – The quality of maximum lucidity of an *intraphysical consciousness,* achieved through recuperation – as far as possible – of his or her cons.

Hyper-thosene *(hyper + tho + sen + ene)* – Heuristic *thosene;* original idea of a discovery; neophilic *thosene;* unit of measurement of invention, according to *Conscientiology.*

Hypnagogy (Greek: *hipnos,* sleep; and *agogos,* conductor) – Transitional twilight condition of *consciousness* between the waking state and natural sleep state. It is an altered state of *consciousness.*

Hypnopompy (Greek: *hipnos,* sleep; and *pompikós,* procession) – A transitional condition of natural sleep, prior to physical awakening. It is a semi-asleep state that precedes the act of waking up. It is characterized by dream images having auditory effects and hallucinatory visions that continue even after waking. It is an altered state of *consciousness.*

Hypo-thosene *(hypo + tho + sen + ene)* – Same as *proto-thosene* or *Phyto-thosene.*

Immanent energy – Primary energy, totally impersonal, neutral and dispersed in all objects or physical creations throughout the universe. It is an omnipotent form, and has still not been mastered by human *consciousness.* It is too subtle to be detected by existing instruments.

Incomplete couple – Couple composed of a man and woman who do not form an intimate couple (a couple that has complete sexual interactions), but who, nevertheless, maintain strong affectionate ties.

Incompletism – Condition wherein a *human consciousness' existential program* is incomplete.

Integrated maturity – State of a more evolved *consciential* maturity beyond biological (physical) or mental (psychological) maturity; *holomaturity.*

Interassistential – Of or pertaining to mutual assistance.

Interassistentiality – The evolutionary necessity for *human consciousnesses* to assist each other through logical, just and mature *interassistential works*.

Intersciential climate – Condition of multiple understanding in an *intersciential* encounter, established through *thosenes* having affinity, especially those *charged* with *consciential energy*. *Intersciential climates* can vary greatly in intensity.

Intersciential intrusion – Action exercised by a consciousness on another.

Interdimensionality – *Intersciential* communication between many *intraphysical* (physical) and *extraphysical* (nonphysical) *dimensions*.

Intermissibility – Quality of the period of intermission between two *intraphysical* lives of a *consciousness*.

Intermission – The *extraphysical* period between 2 of a *consciousness' existential seriations* (*rebirth cycle*).

Intermissive course – Sum total of disciplines and theoretical and practical experiences administered to an *extraphysical consciousness* during its period of *consciential intermission* between two *intraphysical* lives. This course occurs when one has achieved a determinate evolutionary level in one's cycle of personal existences. It has the aim of allowing *consciential completism* in the next *intraphysical life*.

Inter-personal apparition – Appearance of the *consciousness* of a *projector* before *intraphysical consciousnesses*.

Intra-conscientiality – Quality of the specific intimate manifestations of *consciousness*.

Intraphysical consciousness – Human personality; citizen of *intraphysical* society. Outworn synonym: *incarnate*.

Intraphysical euphoria – Euphoria experienced before *somatic* deactivation that is generated through the reasonably satisfactory completion of one's *existential program*, *pre-mortem* euphoria. Ideal condition predisposing one to have a positive *existential moratorium*.

Intraphysical melancholy – Condition of *intraphysical* or *pre-mortem melancholy*.

Intraphysical recycling – An *intraconsciential, existential, intraphysical recycling* or the cerebral renovation of an *in-*

traphysical consciousness through the creation of new synapses (interneural connections) capable of permitting the adjustment of one's *existential program*, the execution of *existential recycling*, *existential inversion*, the acquisition of new ideas, *neo-thosenes*, *hypo-thosenes* and other neophilic conquests of the self-motivated *human consciousness*.

Intraphysical societal virus – Any social *weak* trait in the *intraphysical life* of a *human consciousness*.

Intraphysical society – Society of *intraphysical consciousnesses*; human society.

Intraphysicality – Condition of *intraphysical* or human life, or of the existence of *human consciousness*.

Intra-thosene (*intra + tho + sen + ene*) – *Intraconsciential thosene* of *human consciousness*.

Intrudability – Pathological, *interconsciential thosenic intrusion*. Out-dated equivalent expression: *obsession*. Numerous *intraphysical consciousnesses* are defensive regarding the use of this word.

Intrusive stigma – An evolutionary failure or derailing that is always dramatic and generally pathological, usually stemming from *consciential* self-obsession. This process generates either *intraphysical* or *extraphysical melancholy* and often results in psychic accidents.

Locked existence – Human experience or existential seriation without the production of *conscious projections* (CPs); tropospheric human life having only unconscious, vegetative projections characteristic of the state of evolutionary *extraphysical* coma; locked existential seriation.

Lucid projectability – Lucid, projective paraphysiological quality of *consciousness* capable of provoking the non-alignment of its *holosoma*, through the use of the will, as well as by other means.

Lucidity-recall (a binomial) – Set of two conditions indispensable to the *intraphysical consciousness* for the achievement of a fully satisfactory *lucid projection* outside the body.

Macro-soma (*macro + soma*) – Soma that is *super-customized* for the execution of a specific *existential program*.

Maxi-fraternity – Most evolved, universalist, interconsciential condition that is based on pure fraternity on the part of a *consciousness* who pardons others for transgressions but not him or herself; mega-brotherhood. *Maxi-fraternity* is an inevitable goal in the evolution of all *consciousnesses.*

Maxi-thosene (*maxi* + *tho* + *sen* + *ene*) – *Thosene* peculiar to *Free Consciousnesses.*

Mega-goal – A greater evolutionary objective for a *consciousness.*

Mega-power – The evolved condition of *cosmoethical,* magnum *consciential* lucidity.

Mega-strong trait – The maximal strong trait of a *consciousness.*

Mega-thosene (*mega* + *tho* + *sen* + *ene*) – Same as *orthothosene.*

Mega-weak trait – The maximal weak trait of a *consciousness.*

Mental projective target – Predetermined goal that an *intraphysical consciousness* endeavors to reach using will, intention, mentalization and decision upon noting him or herself lucid while outside the body.

Mentalsoma (*mental* + *soma*) – *Mental body;* extra-*physical body* of discernment of *consciousness.* Plural: *mentalsomas.*

Mentalsomatic cycle – The evolutionary cycle or course that a *consciousness* initiates in its condition of *free consciousness* upon the definitive deactivation of the *psychosoma* (*third death*), consequently living only with the *mentalsoma.*

Mentalsomaticity – Qualities of the manifestations of *intraphysical consciousness* deriving from the *mentalsoma.*

Metasoma (*meta* + *soma*) – Same as *psychosoma,* the *extraphysical* instrument of *extraphysical* and *intraphysical consciousnesses.*

Mini-thosene (*mini* + *tho* + *sen* + *ene*) – *Thosene* of a child, sometimes as a function of their still developing brain.

Mnemonic intrusion – Collision of the intrusive memory of an *extraphysical consciousness* upon the cerebral memory of an *intraphysical consciousness* who has been intruded upon (*para-amnesia*).

Mnemosoma (*mnemo* + *soma*) – The soma when specifically considered in regards to the memory of *consciousness* in all of its forms.

Mono-thanatose – Same as *de-soma*; *first death.*

Mono-thosene (*mono* + *tho* + *sen* + *ene*) – Repetitive *thosene*; fixed idea; mental echo; *re-thosene.*

Morpho-thosene (*morpho* + *tho* + *sen* + *ene*) – A thought or a group of thoughts when gathered together and expressed as having some type of *form.* Archaic expression now fallen out of use: *thought-form.* An accumulation of *morphothosenes* composes a *holothosene.*

Multi-dimensional self-awareness – Condition of lucid maturity of an *intraphysical consciousness* in terms of living a *multi-dimensionally* evolved *consciential* life. This condition is achieved through *lucid projectability.*

Multi-existential cycle – System or condition of continuous alternation – at our current, average evolutionary level – of an *intraphysical* rebirth period (*intraphysical* lifetime or *existential seriation*) followed by an *extraphysical somatic* post-deactivation period or *intermission* (*extraphysical* "lifetime").

Near-Death Experience (NDE) – Involuntary or forced *projection* due to critical circumstances pertaining to a *human consciousness.* NDE is common in cases of terminal illness and survivors of clinical death.

Neophilia – *Intraphysical consciousness'* easy adaptation to new situations, things and occurrences. Opposite of neophobia.

Neo-thosene (*neo* + *tho* + *sen* + *ene*) – *Thosene* of an *intraphysical consciousness* when operating with new synapses or interneural connections – a situation capable of provoking *intraconsciential recycling; unit of measurement* of *consciential* renovation, according to *Conscientiology* or, more appropriately, *Conscientiometry.*

Oneiro-thosene – (*oneiro* + *tho* + *sen* + *ene*) – Dream thosene. Same as *patho-thosene.*

Orgasmic aura (Latin: *aura*, wisp of air)   *Holochakral* energy of *facies sexualis* of a man or woman at the exact moment of sexual orgasm or climax.

Ortho-thosene (*ortho* + *tho* + *sen* + *ene*) – A *just* or *cosmoethical thosene*, pertaining to *consciential holomaturity*, a *unit of measurement* of practical *cosmoethics*, according to *Conscientiometry*.

Pangraphy – Broad, sophisticated multi-modal psychic writing.

Para – Prefix that signifies *beyond* or *beside*, as in *parabrain*. Also signifies *extraphysical*.

Para-brain – *Extraphysical* brain of the *psychosoma* of a *consciousness* in the *extraphysical* (*extraphysical consciousness*), *intraphysical* (*intraphysical consciousness*), and *projected* states.

Para-genetics – Genetics of a human embryo submitted to the influence of *consciential* inheritance from the previous life through the *psychosoma*.

Para-man – *Extraphysical consciousness* having the appearance of a man or projected man. Outworn synonymous expression: *masculine spiritual entity*.

Para-pathology – Pathology of the vehicles of manifestation of *consciousness*, excluding the human body or *soma*.

Para-physiology – Physiology of the vehicles of manifestation of *consciousness*, excluding the human body or *soma*.

Parapsychophysical repercussions – Reactions between 2 vehicles of *consciential* manifestation when they enter into contact with each other. They can be different vehicles of the same *consciousness* or similar vehicles of 2 or more *consciousnesses*. These repercussions can be *intraphysical* and *extraphysical*.

Para-thosene (*para* + *tho* + *sen* + *ene*) – *Thosene* of an *extraphysical consciousness*.

Para-woman – *Extraphysical consciousness* having the appearance of a woman or projected woman. Outworn synonymous expression: *feminine spiritual entity*.

Passes-to-the-dark – Popular expression signifying the daily, technical transmission of *consciential energies* by an *intraphysical consciousness*, directly to *extraphysical consciousnesses* and *projected intraphysical consciousnesses*. This is performed in the waking state with continuous assistance from the. Technical expression: *penta* (personal energetic task).

Patho-thosene (*patho* + *tho* + *sen* + *ene*) – Pathological *thosene* or a thosene of *consciential* dementia; *little venial sin*; sick intention; *cerebral rumination*.

Penial aura – *Sex-chakral* energy around the penis, notably when in erection, perceivable by any motivated individual, especially by the sexually excited man.

Penta (*pe* + *en* + *ta*) – Multi-dimensional, daily, *personal energetic task*. The individual who performs *penta* receives continuous assistance from the *Helpers* on a long-term basis or for the rest of their life. Popular expression: *passes-to-the-dark*.

Personal experience – Non-transferable, direct, personal experimentation by an *intraphysical consciousness* who is on his or her evolutionary path.

Personal principles – Package of guiding values and initiatives of *consciential* life, chosen by a *consciousness* through *holomaturity*, multi-dimensionality and day-to-day *cosmoethicality*.

Phenomenon concomitant to CP – That phenomenon occurring, whether within the time-space *continuum* or not, simultaneously with a *conscious projection*, in a spontaneous or unexpected manner.

Physical base – Safe locale, chosen by the *intraphysical consciousness* to leave his or her *soma* in repose while consciously projected to another, exterior, *consciential* dimension; *duodrome*. A domiciliary *projectiogenic holothosene*. Has a direct relation to: energetically sealed bedroom; *penta*; *consciential epicenter*; *extraphysical clinic*; *projectarium*; *precognitarium*; *retrocognitarium*.

Phyto-thosene (*phyto* + *tho* + *sen* + *ene*) – The rudimentary *thosene* of a plant; the *lexical unit* of a plant, according to *Conscientiology*.

Podo-soma (*podo* + *soma*) – The *soma* when considered specifically in regards to the application of feet or foot-related work, as in the case of a soccer player.

Poly-karma (*poly* + *karma*) – Principle of cause and effect active in evolution of *consciousness*, when centered in an experience of cosmic *maxi-fraternity*, beyond *ego-karma* and *group-karma*.

Poly-karmality – Qualities of the *poly-karmic* manifestations of *consciousness.*

Post-somatic intermission – A *consciousness'* *extraphysical* period immediately following its *somatic* deactivation.

Precognitarium – Physical base technically prepared for the production of precognitive CPs.

Pre-couple – Preliminary stage in human sexuality within *intraphysical society;* flirting.

Pre-intraphysical mandate – *Existential program* for human life, planned before the *intraphysical* rebirth of a *consciousness; existential program.*

Pre-kundalini – Secondary chakra at the sole of the foot. There are 2 *pre-kundalini* chakras in the *holosoma* of an *intraphysical consciousness* – one on the bottom of each foot. This is a *conscientiological* expression.

Pre-serenissimus – *Intraphysical* or *extraphysical consciousness* who does not yet live a life of lucid *serenism* (see *Homo sapiens serenissimus).*

Pre-somatic intermission – A *consciousness' extraphysical* period immediately preceding its *intraphysical* rebirth.

Primo-thosene (*primo + tho + sen + ene*) – Same as the *First* C*ause of the universe;* the first compound thought. This term has no plural form.

Projectarium – *Physical base* technically prepared for the production of consciousness projections.

Projectio-critique – *Projectiological* critique.

Projectiography – Technical study of *projectiological* records.

Projectiology (Latin: *projectio,* projection; Greek: *logos,* treatise) – Science that studies *projection of consciousness* and its effects, as well as the projection of *consciential energies* outside the *holosoma.*

Projectiotherapy – Science of prophylaxis and therapies derived from *projectiological* research and techniques.

Projective phenomenon – A specific psychic occurrence within the scope of *projectiological* research.

Projective recess – Existential phase of an *intraphysical consciousness* characterized by a spontaneous cessation – almost always temporary –within a sequence of intensive lucid projective experiences.

Proto-thosene (*proto + tho + sen + ene*) – More rudimentary *thosene;* same as *phyto-thosene* or *hypo-thosene.*

Psychic accident – Physical or psychological disturbance generated through energetic, *interconsciential* or pathological influences, generally having an *extraphysical* or multi-dimensional origin.

Psychic signs – Self-aware existence, identification and employment of energetic, animic, psychic and personal signs that all *intraphysical consciousnesses* possess.

Psychosoma (Greek: *psyche,* soul; *soma,* body) – *Emotional para-body* of *consciousness;* the *objective body* of *intraphysical consciousness.*

Psychosomatic intrusion – Invasion of a *consciousness* by another through emotionality, or through the *psychosoma.*

Rethosene (*re + tho + sen + ene*) – Repeated thosene. Same as *monothosene* or fixed idea.

Retrocognitarium – *Physical base* technically prepared for the production of *retrocognitive conscious projections (CPs).*

Retrocognition (Latin: *retro,* back; *cognoscere,* to know) – Perceptive capacity whereby an *intraphysical consciousness* knows facts, scenes forms, objects, successes and experiences that pertain to a time in the distant past. These issues commonly have to do with his or her *holo-memory.*

Retrothosene (*retro + tho + sen + ene*) – *Thosene* specifically related to *self-retrocognitions;* same as the engram of mnemotechnics; the *unit of measurement* of *retrocognitions,* according to *Conscientiometry.*

Self-conscientiality – Quality of level of self-knowledge of a *consciousness;* mega-knowledge.

Self-projection – The intentional or willful departure of the *intraphysical consciousness* to another *consciential* dimension, utilizing the *psychosoma* or the *mentalsoma.*

Self-thosene (*self + tho + sen + ene*) – *Thosene* of the *consciousness* itself.

Self-unrelenting – *Intraphysical consciousness* who does not pardon his or her own errors or omissions, in order to eliminate conscious self-corruption. This positive state supports the likewise healthy condition of *hetero*-forgiver, a sincere *universal forgiver* of all beings forever – *a basic principle of mega-brotherhood.*

Semi-conscious projection (SCP) – Dream experience in which a projected *intraphysical consciousness* finds him or herself lucid to some degree, in a confused manner; lucid dream. It is not an ideal *projection of consciousness.*

Sene (*sen* + *ene*) – Sentiment and *consciential energy.*

Serenissimus – Popular name for *Homo sapiens serenissimus.*

Seriality – Quality of *consciousness* submitted to *existential seriation* (rebirth cycle*).*

Sex-chakra (*sex* + *chakra*) – Root or *sexual chakra of human consciousness.* Ancient expression related to the *consciential energy* of this chakra: *kundalini* (*serpentine fire*).

Sex-soma (*sex* + *soma*) – The *soma* when considered specifically in relation to its sex.

Sex-somatics – Study of the *soma,* specifically in regards to its sex or sex-soma and its relationship to *intraphysical consciousness,* whether man or woman.

Sex-thosene (*sex* + *tho* + *sen* + *ene*) – Sexual fantasy; the *unit of measurement* of mental adultery, according to *Conscientiometry.*

Sleep – Natural state of rest in man and in higher animals that is especially characterized by the periodic, normal suppression of perceptive activity, voluntary motor functions, and the act of relating to life. This occurs through the relaxation of the senses and muscles, reduction in cardiac and respiratory frequencies, and continues during dream activity. The organism recuperates from physical fatigue during sleep.

Soma – Human body; body of an individual in the *Animal* kingdom, *Chordata* phylum, *Mammiferous* class, *Primates* order, *Hominidae* family, *Homo* genus, and *Homo sapiens* species – being the most elevated level of animal on this planet; the most rudimentary vehicle of the *holosoma* of *human consciousness,* regardless of its appearance.

Spermatic intrusion – Introduction of a man's sperm into a woman's *sex-soma* during the sex act.

Strong trait – Strong point or trait of the personality of an *intraphysical consciousness*; positive component of the structure of one's *consciential* universe that propels the evolution of *consciousness*.

Sub-thosene (*sub* + *tho* + *sen* + *ene*) – *Thosene* charged with *consciential energy* from the *abdominal sub-brain*, most notably energy of the *umbilical-chakra*; the *unit of measurement* of the *abdominal sub-brain*, according to *Conscientiometry*.

Suspended animation – That state in which an *intraphysical consciousness* has temporarily suspended the essential vital functions of its cellular body, later returning to its normal physiological conditions. In certain cases, this occurs without suffering any damage to personal health – the cells surviving in a metabolism of human hibernation.

Sympathetic assimilation – Willful assimilation (absorption) of the *consciential energies* of another *consciousness*, resulting from a degree of openness or rapport with said *consciousness*. Not uncommonly, this condition is accompanied by the decodification of a set of another *consciousness'* *thosenes*.

Sympathetic de-assimilation – Cessation of the *sympathetic assimilation* of *consciential energies* through the use of one's will, normally through the installation of a *vibrational state*.

Tachy-thosene (*tachy* + *tho* + *sen* + *ene*) – Rapid thosene, natural to the *tachy-psychic* (quick thinking) *intraphysical consciousness*.

Tele-thosene (*tele* + *tho* + *sen* + *ene*) – Same as *homothosene*.

Theorice (*theor* + *ice*) – Experience of both theory and practice on the part of an *intraphysical* or *extraphysical consciousness*.

Thosen (*tho* + *sen*) – Thought and sentiment.

Thosene (*tho* + *sen* + *ene*) – Practical unit of manifestation of *consciousness*, according to *Conscientiology*, that considers thought or idea (conception), sentiment or emotion, and *consciential energy* as being 3 indissociable elements.

Thosener – Instrument through which *consciousness* manifests its thoughts and acts. In the case of *intraphysical consciousness*, the fundamental thosener is the *soma*.

Thosenic intrusion – Invasion of a *consciousness* upon another by way of the *mentalsoma*.

Thosenity – Quality of one's *thosenic* awareness.

Tri-thanatose – Deactivation and discarding of the *psychosoma* upon the entrance of *Homo sapiens serenissimus* into the condition of *Free Consciousness; third death; third de-soma*.

Umbilical-chakra (*umbilical* + *chakra*) – Chakra located above the navel. Related to the (abdominal) physiology and paraphysiology of *human consciousness*.

Universalism – Set of ideas derived from the universality of the basic laws of nature and the universe. Universalism inevitably becomes the dominant philosophy of consciousness, as a result of our natural evolution; cosmism.

Vehicle of consciousness – Instrument or body whereby *consciousness* manifests in *intraphysicality* (*intraphysical consciousness*) and in the *extraphysical* dimensions (projected individual and *extraphysical consciousness*).

Verbaction (*verb* + *action*) – Coherent interaction between what is said and done by a *consciousness*; result of one's words being ratified by one's actions.

Vibrational state – Technical condition of maximal dynamization of the *holochakral* energies, through the impulse of will.

Waking non-alignment – Psychic condition in which the *intraphysical projector*, while in the ordinary waking state, perceives that the *psychosoma* is in *non-alignment* or not completely reintegrated with the *soma*. This generates the intensification of psychic perceptions and energetic and psychic phenomena.

Weak trait – Weak point or trait of the personality of an *intraphysical consciousness*; negative component of the structure of one's *consciential* universe that the individual is not yet able to overcome.

Willful intrusion – Invasion of the will of a *consciousness* on another through hetero-suggestion or hetero-hypnosis.

Xenophrenia (Greek: *xenos*, strange; *phrem*, mind) – State of *human consciousness* outside the normal pattern of waking state, induced by physical, physiological, psychological, pharmacological or psychic agents; altered state of *consciousness.*

Xeno-thosene *xeno + tho + sen + ene*) – Meddlesome *thosene* of an *intruder* in the occurrences of *thosenic intrusion, mental wedge, unit of measurement* of *interconsciential intrusion,* according to *Conscientiometry.*

Zoo-thosene (*zoo + tho + sen + ene*) – *Thosene* of an unaware sub-human animal; *unit of measurement* of a sub-human animal's *consciential* principle, according to *Conscientiometry.*

ABBREVIATIONS

Observations: The following is a list of abbreviations used in *Projectiology* and *Conscientiology* texts.

A.D. = anno Domini (Latin: in the year of the Lord)
add. = address
AIDS = Acquired Immune Deficiency Syndrome
alph. = alphabetized index of subjects
app. = appendix(es)
B.C. = before Christ
B.O. = body odor
bibl. = bibliography
bio. = biography
br. = brochure
CD = compact disk
CD-ROM = compact disk read-only memory
CE = *consciential energy*
chap. = chapter
Chin. = Chinese
chs. = chapters
CIPRO = International Congress of Projectiology
cm. = centimeter(s)
Co. = company
collab. = collaboration
comm. = commentator
CP = *conscious projection* or *consciential projection.* Can be lucid, semi-lucid or unconscious.
Dan. = Danish
def. = definition
dic. = dictionary
Du. = Dutch language
ed. = edition
eds. = editions
EHE = Exceptional Human Experience
elec. = electricity
Elvis = to be dead (in war)
ene = *consciential energy*

Engl. = English language
epil. = epilogue
esp. = extrasensory perception
Esper. = Esperanto language
etc. = et cetera (and so forth)
ex. = example
exx. = examples
FAO = Food and Agriculture Organization
FC = *free consciousness*
fig. = figure
figs. = figures
Fr. = French language
geo. = reference to geography
Ger. = German language
gloss. = glossary
Gr. = Greek language
hi-fi = high-fidelity; type of apparatus for producing sound recordings or reproductions.
hr = human resources (personnel department of a company)
ICU = intensive-care unit (of a hospital).
IE = *immanent energy*
IIPC = International Institute of Projectiology and Projectiology
ill. = illustration
in. = inch(es)
INAMPS = *Instituto Nacional de Assistencia Medica e Previdencia Social*; National Institute of Medical Assistance and Social Welfare.
INAN = *Instituto Nacional de Alimentação e Nutricção*; National Institute of Alimentation and Nutrition.
indig. = indigenous
intro. = introduction
IQ = Intelligence Quotient
It. = Italian language
Jpn. = Japanese language
Lat. = Latin language
lb. = pound
lbs. = pounds
LP = lucid projectability
LSD = Lysergic Acid Diethylamide

m. = meter(s)
mg. = milligram(s)
n. = number(s)
NDE = Near-Death Experience
ngo = Non-governmental Organization
OBE = Out-of-Body Experience; extracorporeal experience.
ono. = onomastic index; list of proper names
OOBE = Out-of-the-Body Experience.
PE = personal experience
PEE = personal extraphysical experience
PEEs = personal extraphysical experiences
PEs = personal experiences
pg. = page
PK = psychokinesis; psychic phenomena and physical effects.
pmr = progressive muscular relaxation
Port. = Portuguese language
pseud. = pseudonym
questn. = questionnaire
refs. = bibliographic reference
relig. = religious
Rus. = Russian language
Sansk. = Sanskrit language.
SC = *somatic consciousness*
sci-fi = science-fiction
SCP = semi-conscious projection
SCPs = semi-conscious projections
Sen = sentiment or emotion.
Sene = sentiment and consciential energy
Sp. = Spanish language
St. = Saint
Syn. = synonym
tab. = table
tabs. = tables
Tho = thought or idea
Thosen = thought and idea
trans. = translator
transc. = transcription
TV = television
U.S.A. = United States of America

UFO = unidentified flying object
UN = United Nations.
UNESCO = United Nations Educational, Scientific and Cultural Organization.
UNICEF = United Nations International Children's Emergency Fund.
UP = unconscious projection
vol. = volume(s)
VS = *vibrational state*
WHO = World Heath Organization.
WIA = wounded in action.

BIBLIOGRAPHY

1. VIEIRA, Waldo; *Miniglossário da Conscienciologia*; 57 p.; 17 x 11 cm.; Spiral bound; 1st edition; Rio de Janeiro, RJ, Brazil; International Institute of Projectiology; 1992; pg. 54.

2. IDEM; *O Que é a Conscienciologia*; 180 pp.; 100 chpts.; 3 refs.; glos. 280 terms; alph.; 21x14 cm.; br.; 1st edition; Rio de Janeiro, RJ, Brazil; International Institute of Projectiology; 1994; pgs. 30, 72, 107, 139, 156, 160, 168, 173.

3. IDEM; *Projeciologia: Panorma das Experiências da Consciência Fora do Corpo Humano*; XXVIII + 900p.; 475 chs.; 40 illus.; 1,907 refs.; gloss. 15 terms; ono.; geo.; alph.; 27 x 18.5 x 5 cm.; enc. 3rd edition; Londri; Parana; Brazil; Livraria e Editora Universalista; 1990; pgs. 389-393.

4. IDEM; *Projections of the Consciousness: A Diary of Out-of-Body Experiences*; 224 p.; glos. 25 terms; alph.; 21 x 14 cm; br.; 1st edition revised; Rio de Janeiro, RJ, Brazil; International Institute of Projectiology; 1995; pg. 153-155.

5. IDEM; 700 Experimentos da Conscienciologia; 1058 pgs.; 700 chs.; 300 tests; 8 indexes; 2 tables; 600 numbered enumerations; ono; 5,116 refs.; geo.; gloss.; 280 terms; alph.; 28.5 x 21.5 x 7 cm.; enc.; 1st edition; Rio de Janeiro, RJ, Brazil; International Institute of Projectiology; 1994; pgs. 171, 178, 180, 183, 198, 242, 283, 322, 352, 353, 355, 409, 412, 424, 431, 432, 468, 484, 539, 542, 564, 572, 580, 595, 671, 672, 693, 700, 726, 736, 737, 739, 741, 759.

INDEX

Observation: The numbers listed are page numbers. In the cases
of there being more than one page number, the one in italic indicates the main reference.

142

| International Institute of Projectiology and Conscientiology |

The International Institute of Projectiology and Conscientiology (IIPC) is a non-profit institution of research and education, or laboratory-school, that has been dedicated to the study of consciousness and its bioenergetic and projective (out-of-body) manifestations since its foundation in 1988. Having the objective of disseminating its Conscientiology and Projectiology research findings to researchers and the public, IIPC has published various books and has developed a regular program of educational activities, conferences, courses, lectures, workshops and other activities at all of its offices. Groups of foreigners regularly visit the Institute, which is able to give its courses in Portuguese, English, Spanish and French.

IIPC Statistics

Offices:
- Main office in Rio de Janeiro
- 63 national and international offices: Alfenas, Americana, Aracaju, Arapiraca, Avare, Belem, Belo Horizonte, Blumenau, Brasília, Buenos Aires, Campo Grande, Cascavel, Criciúma, Cuiabá, Curitiba, Feira de Santana, Florianópolis, Fortaleza, Iguacu Falls, Goiânia, Guaira, Guarapuava, Guaratingueta, Ijui, Itajuba, Ji-Parana, Joinville, João Pessoa, Jundiaí, Lambari, Lisbon, London, Londrina, Maceió, Manaus, Maringá, Mogi das Cruzes, Mogi-Guaçu, Montes Claros, Miami, Natal, Niteroi, New York, Novo Hamburgo, Osasco, Pelotas, Pirassununga, Porto Alegre, Porto Velho, Recife, Riberão Preto, Rio Branco, Salvador, Santos, São Bernardo do Campo, São José dos Campos, São Paulo, São Pedro D'Aldeia, São Vicente, Torres, Três Pontas, Vila Mariana, Vitória.

28 Research Groups in 6 Areas:
- Computer Science
- Conscientiological Intraphysical Society
- Conscientiotherapy

- Existential Inversion
- Existential Recycling
- Leading-edge Research

Mailing List:
- 70,000 Individuals
- 1,275 Institutions

Educational activities. IIPC has developed two types of courses:

Regular courses include those with and without prerequisite. The five stages (in English) with prerequisite provide information on the history, ideas and research results achieved over the last 30 years in the field of Conscientiology and Projectiology, as well as teaching and allowing practice with various techniques. Non-prerequisite courses focus on specific themes in the area of Conscientiology and Projectiology.

Extracurricular courses, also without prerequisite, are a result of the research performed by IIPC teachers in diverse fields of study in conventional science, as well as Conscientiology and Projectiology, with a consciential approach. Human sexuality, existential inversion and penta (personal energetic task) are among the themes addressed.

Lectures, open to the public and free of charge, are held weekly at all IIPC offices.

IIPC International Offices

Buenos Aires, Argentina
Since 1992, the Buenos Aires office has operated as a base serving to integrate Conscientiology and Projectiology in South American countries, as well as the rest of Latin America.

Lisbon, Portugal
The Lisbon office has been offering its activities since 1994 and maintains contact with researchers and organizations in Spain, France and Italy.

London, UK
The London office gives the CDP on a regular basis and maintains contact with the Society for Psychical Research (SPR) – the mother organization of the ASPR.

Ottawa, Canada
The newly activated Ottawa office holds public lectures and offers the CDP on a regular basis.

New York & Miami, USA
The New York and Miami offices have been giving the IIPC Consciousness Development Program (CDP) in English since 1994. The New York office currently offers the CDP in New York, New Jersey and Massachusetts. It maintains contact with various institutions, including the American Society for Psychical Research (ASPR), one of the oldest and most important parapsychology research institutions in the world. The Miami office, established in 1994, holds its activities in English and Spanish.

Having the multi-dimensional and cosmoethical objective of catalyzing the holomaturity of more aware pre-serenissimus, IIPC is open to all researchers who are motivated to collaborate with its advanced proposals. If you are interested in working as a mini-piece of the maxi-mechanism of conscientiality, contact the IIPC office closest to you.

Headquarters
R. Visconde de Pirajá, 572 / 6° andar – Ipanema – Rio de Janeiro – RJ – Brasil – CEP 22410-002
Fone (5521) 512.9229 – Fax (5521) 512.4735
Internet: E-mail: iip@ax.ibase.org.br
Home Page: http://www.ibase.org.br/~iip

Buenos Aires, Argentina
Calle Azcuenaga, 797 / 10°A
Pc. Buenos Aires 1029 - Argentina
Tel./fax: (541) 951-5048

Lisbon, Portugal
Rua Pascoal de Melo, 84 - 1° Esq. sl.11
Lisbon 1000 - Portugal
 Tel: (511) 353-6339
E-mail: iippt@tpone.telepac.pt

London, UK
34 Waterbank Rd.
Catford, London SE6 3DH, UK
Tel.: (181) 698-9449
E-mail: iipuk@dillons.co.uk

Ottawa, Canada
60 Laurie Court
Kanata, ONT K2L 1S4, Canada
Tel./fax: (613) 831-4483
E-mail: asalgado@magi.com

Miami, USA
7800 S.W. 57 Ave., Suite 207D
South Miami, FL 33143, USA
Tel./fax: (305) 668-4668
E-mail: iipusafl@aol.com

New York, USA
20 East 49 Street, Suite 2F
New York, NY 10017 USA
Tel./fax: (718) 721-6257
E-mail: iipnyusa@aol.com

For information on other offices, contact IIPC's main office.

Conscientiological Complex

The International Institute of Projectiology and Conscientiology (IIPC) is implanting a *CONSCIENTIOLOGICAL COMPLEX* in Iguacu Falls, Paraná, Brazil. This will be a center for work, research, residence and *conscientiological* assistance. An area of 24.2 acres (9.68 hectares) will be developed. This area is next to natural foliage and a stream. Its objective is the implantation of a center for the research and dissemination of the worthy ideas of *conscientiology* and *projectiology*, as a type of *conscientiological* district. One of the characteristics of the area of Iguacu Falls is its great quantity of high quality *immanent energy* – a fact which greatly aids in the *holothosene* of this future district. Iguacu Falls also stands out due to its proximity to Argentina and Paraguay. It is the second largest touristic area in Brazil and, for this reason, receives a great quantity of visitors from the world over. These characteristics of Iguacu Falls contribute towards the globalization of the *clarification task* – promoted by IIP. The *Conscientiological Complex* is composed of the following facets:

Center for Higher Studies of Consciousness.

The *Center for Higher Studies of Consciousness* is the Complex's research center. Its objective is to promote social benefits through educational, scientific, technological, commercial and ethical solutions, accelerating *group evolution.*

The following spaces are planned:

- The *Projectarium* is a building that combines all ideal elements characteristic for the engendering of lucid projection of consciousness.

- The *Holo-repository* is a display facility for the permanent exposition of artifacts of knowledge that will be distributed among 100 stands and will include space for Dr. Vieira's library, which includes 30,000 volumes, being one of the most specialized in the world on subjects regarding projection of consciousness.

- Immersion Courses, or Extension in Conscientiology/Projectiology 1 (ECP1) and Extension in Conscientiology/Projectiology 2 (ECP2), that are given over weekends and require exclusive accommodations.

- Conscientiotherapy (consciousness therapy) Clinic, for public consultations.

- Event Pavilion – a large building in which all IIPC activities are concentrated, such as congresses, forums, symposiums, conferences workshops, assemblies, video and film projections, etc.

- Lodging for researchers – a hotel service for those engaged in the activities of the Center.

- Publishing House and Print Shop for the literary production of the Complex and IIPC.

- Conscientiological School, allowing individuals to work according to cosmoethical and universalist principles.

- Environmental Recuperation of the entire area, including a wooded area comprising 20% of the total area of the Center. This area will be devoted to planting fruit-bearing, medicinal and bird-attracting plants, forest recuperation and landscaping with native plant species.

- Conscientiological Administration – a building that would join the teams that will administrate the Complex. These teams will also offer administrative assistance to interested professional companies.

The Center's plans include innovative principles, aiming to increase the researchers' effectiveness, focusing on *mentalsomatics*. The *holo-repository* is the central building of this project.

Conscientiological Residential Complex. Adapted to the profile of the *conscientiology/projectiology* researcher, this residential complex has a tone of multi-dimensional architecture that takes *holosomatic* and *multi-dimensional* aspects into consideration. It is planned with the intention of creating a residential complex similar to advanced *extraphysical communities*, having a sensible philosophy and space planning. The residents will have areas for performing *penta*, research, maintaining a library, etc. This complex will catalyze group and individual existential programs and allow the residents to work in an environment of heightened conviviality. This tends to predispose those individuals engaged in this mega-challenge to an inevitably greater self-knowledge, and an unprecedented self-confrontation within a group of persons interested in evolution of consciousness.

Service Shopping Center. In order to completely meet the needs of the Complex's researchers, the service shopping center was conceived within the philosophical principles of *conscientiology*. Its aim is to bring together *conscientiological* companies and professionals who will offer *cosmoethical* services to the general public.